THE AUTISTIC SLEUTH

Screen Portrayals of Detectives on the Spectrum in Sherlock Holmes Adaptations, The Millennium Trilogy, The Bridge, Death Note, The Curious Incident of the Dog in the Night-Time, and Other Productions.

By Chris Chan

With Patricia Meyer Chan, Ph.D.

© Copyright 2024
Chris Chan and Dr. Patricia Meyer Chan

The right of Chris Chan and Dr. Patricia Meyer Chan to be identified as the authors of this work has been asserted by them in accordance with the Copyright, Designs and Patents Act 1998.

All rights reserved. No reproduction, copy or transmission of this publication may be made without express prior written permission. No paragraph of this publication may be reproduced, copied or transmitted except with express prior written permission or in accordance with the provisions of the Copyright Act 1956 (as amended). Any person who commits any unauthorised act in relation to this publication may be liable to criminal prosecution and civil claims for damage.

All characters appearing in this work are fictitious. Any resemblance to real persons, living or dead, is purely coincidental. The opinions expressed herein are those of the author and not of MX Publishing.

Hardcover ISBN 978-1-80424-468-5
Paperback ISBN 978-1-80424-469-2
ePub ISBN 978-1-80424-470-8
PDF ISBN 978-1-80424-471-5

Published by MX Publishing
335 Princess Park Manor, Royal Drive,
London, N11 3GX
www.mxpublishing.co.uk
Cover design by Awan

Once more to my parents: my father, Dr. Carlyle Chan, and my mother and co-author, Dr. Patricia Meyer Chan.

And to my godmother, Jeanette Kirchner, whose help and support have been invaluable.

TABLE OF CONTENTS

Introduction – Autism, Crime Dramas, and Understanding   1
Chapter 1 – How Mysteries Taught Me How to Connect with Other People   7
Chapter 2 – A Collection of Potentially Autistic Fictional Sleuths   31
Chapter 3 – Autism: The Condition That Must Not Be Named   66
Chapter 4 – How Realistic is "Realism?"   77
Chapter 5 – Autism: Born or Made?   82
Chapter 6 – Wardrobe Functions   100
Chapter 7 – Visual Representations of Mental Processes and Observation   111
Chapter 8 – Love, Sex, and Autism   121
Chapter 9 – But You've Got to Have Friends   148
Chapter 10 – The Autistic Perpetrator   159
Chapter 11 – Looking Through an Autistic Lens   191
Conclusion – Personal Perspectives, Connections, and Suggestions for Improvement   203
Appendix: 12 Things to Know About Parishioners with Autism   210
Bibliography   219

INTRODUCTION– Autism, Crime Dramas, and Understanding

This book was written to help people with autism put their mental processes and experiences into words, and to assist neurotypical individuals with understanding what life may be like for the autistic. Over the past few decades, autism, once a narrowly defined and rarely studied condition, has entered the cultural mainstream. As the definition of autism has expanded and grown more nuanced in the wake of increased research, it is not surprising that the entertainment industry has increased its focus on this mental condition as well.

But for all of the newfound public awareness of autism, the ability to convey what it is, beyond a cold and clinical list of diagnostic criteria, remains elusive. Too often, stereotypes, broad generalities, and oversimplifications have stood in the way of explaining what it is like to filter the world through an autistic mind. Additionally, while much valuable research has been done, scientific papers are generally presented through academic lenses and mental health professional jargon. Certainly there is nothing inherently wrong with conveying the results of studying autism in such a manner, but the consequence of addressing autism through a dispassionate scientific approach is that it overlooks the emotional factor. There is a great chasm between identifying the characteristics of autism, and conveying what it is like to actually experience autism.

It is often noted that no one really knows if one sees colors in the same way that other people do. It is impossible to say with any degree of certainty that another person's eyes process red, for example, precisely the same way as someone else. It's certainly possible that someone else might see a slightly lighter or darker shade than someone else, and there's no way to really describe the color through words, especially when one cannot be sure if someone else shares the same conception of "cherry," "candy apple," or "crimson" as another person. There is no way to set a universal benchmark.

So it is with autism. Words are often painfully inadequate to explain certain facets of autism, such as meltdowns, responses to stimuli, and reactions to memories. Sometimes the mere attempt to verbalize the intensity of the feelings a person with autism can experience can bring on an intense reaction, perhaps an involuntary emotional or physical response, possibly "stimming," or a full-fledged meltdown with embarrassing effects. Terms like "painful" or "overwhelming" are evocative, but insufficiently detailed as to duplicate an experience. Dramatic portrayals of people with autism, including those that use stylized depictions in order to demonstrate the mental workings of their subjects, are a useful comparative device, though they must be used with caution.

Actors portraying the autistic are often a very blunt tool for describing how real-life people with autism feel. The varieties of autistic experience are so vast and unique that what might be an uncannily accurate reproduction of one autistic person's mind could be utterly unlike what another person with autism feels. In many ways, many of the most prominent actor portrayals of people on the spectrum (or more often than not, debatably autistic) are a useful tool to explain certain autistic reactions.

But because the autism spectrum is so vast, much of what is shown in films and television either provides an incomplete picture, or fails to illustrate how a specific example is not necessarily universal, or even representative of a majority. Many of the portrayals discussed here have been criticized for not being "realistic" or "accurate" treatments of autism. Based on personal experience, I have found that some of the leading depictions that have been most fiercely attacked on the grounds of correctness are indeed true-to-life, but only for certain people with autism, like me.

I wrote this book because in many cases, what I saw on television was an unsettlingly similar duplication of my own mental experiences, though in many respects far from identical. It is my belief that in the decades to come, as autism is further researched and more people with autism give voice to their experiences, the complexities of the spectrum will be better explored, and diagnoses will be more narrowly and separately categorized. It is my opinion that in the future, different forms of autism will be labelled as comparable but distinct branches. What names will be given to those types will be anybody's guess. "Asperger's," the particular branch of autism with which I was initially diagnosed, has fallen out of favor, partially due to the background of the man for which it is named, and now the umbrella term "autism spectrum disorder" is currently used. I would not be surprised if other name changes were to follow in the future, especially with some people's discomfort over the use of the word "disorder." Currently, terminology like Autism Spectrum Disorder Level 1, 2, and 3, denoting the increasing severity of symptoms, is being used to clarify the severity of issues people with autism have, but this categorization may be revised as well in the future.

The wording used to describe autism has evolved a lot over the years, and it will continue to change in the decades to come. When I was officially diagnosed in 2009, the term used to describe my condition was Asperger's Syndrome. Within a few years, the American Psychological Association decided to discontinue the use of that term, eliminating Asperger's as an official diagnostic term and replacing it with the general term of autism.

Officially, "autism" is short for "autism spectrum disorder," but this term is itself controversial, because many people, including myself, take offense to the use of the word "disorder." Certainly some people with autism suffer from it, and in many cases the overstimulation and meltdowns and other negative effects cause a disability, but to call autism itself a disorder is to denigrate the autistic mind, and it is certainly not always the case that if the option existed, people with autism would choose to have their brains changed into neurotypical ones.

There is also a debate over the ordering of words. Some people argue that "autistic people" makes autism the first and most central character of a person, whereas "people with autism" makes the subject being described a human being first and makes the autism secondary. There are opposing views on this, especially due to the fact that "people with autism" can often come across as clunky. Often, due to needing to create better-flowing prose, I will switch back and forth between this terminology.

It is not just terms that cause controversy. Symbols are comparably divisive. For a while, popular symbols for autism featured jigsaw puzzle pieces, often of different colors. As a fan of jigsaw puzzles, I liked this symbolism, but it fell out of favor when other people with autism argued that the imagery creates the impression that the autistic are childlike and obsessed with making things fit their preferred patterns. I can understand that perspective, and I certainly do not want anybody to feel marginalized by a symbol meant to represent them. The current, most prominent symbol for autism is a multicolored eternity symbol, symbolizing the diversity of the autism spectrum. Some people who deal with serious problems due to their autism find a depressing ominousness in the eternity symbol, as if it is saying that their troubles will never end, so the longevity of the eternity symbol as a representation of the autistic may be shorter than its creators hoped. No term or symbol is perfect, and most of them have unexpected implications.

I have no doubt that if people are still reading this book in twenty years, that some of the terminology will be considered outdated, even offensive. I can assure readers that no intention of causing insult is meant, and that at the time of writing I am trying to use the official or most widely accepted terminology, but just because I use these terms, I do not believe that they are necessarily the best and most descriptive words. When "Asperger's" was widely used, it referred to a specific form of autism, arguably a subset of the autistic spectrum. Like many people, I found "Asperger's" to be more descriptive, as this diagnosis highlighted particular attributes, and personally, I have a deep attachment to the term, as it was a great relief to me to have a widely accepted term to describe a condition that had previously been misdiagnosed with much more ominous terminology. I would not be surprised if "autism spectrum disorder" is ultimately dubbed too broad and vague, and that more specialized terms for different forms of autism will be developed in the future. I do think that Asperger's would be a more descriptive term, well-suited for most of the detectives discussed in this book. But for various understandable reasons, including the personal life and political affiliations of Hans Asperger, the term has been phased out, and I am minimizing its use here. When the word "Asperger's" is used on the show or film, or in a comment by someone connected to the show, it will be used here.

I am trying to use the best terminology possible for this study, though I still have concerns that many of these words will become dated in the future. All I am trying to do is use the best, least controversial, and most widely effective terminology to discuss the growing phenomenon of detectives with autism (or at least, have certain autistic characteristics) in film and television.

This book does not intend to castigate or dismiss any of the characters and screenplays discussed here, but it will try to reframe critical perspectives and place any lessons or messages expressed in them into broader context.

There is one point that I need to address. Recently, when a series of my articles were posted on a blog, one commenter brought to my attention that there is another person who uses the same name as mine, who also identifies as having autism. I am not the individual known for YouTube videos, and I have used the name "Chris Chan" professionally for decades. My name is fairly common, and I write under the name "Chris Chan" instead of "Christopher Chan" or "Christopher M. Chan" because there are so many other people in various fields who write under those names. For a while I considered using a totally unique pseudonym, but I prefer to write under my own name, and I was inspired by the late, great children's television host Mr. Fred Rogers, who dealt with awkward rumors about being a sniper in the Vietnam War for decades because there was a soldier with the same name. I figure that if Mr. Rogers can deal with that kind of confusion and still maintain his own public persona, I can too.

Hopefully, this book will give people ideas as to how to better communicate with others and understand other experiences. And to better explain the perspective with which I analyze these crime shows, I have to begin by talking about my own mind...

–Chris Chan

CHAPTER ONE
How Mysteries Taught Me How to Connect with Other People

(Note: This chapter is a revised version of my lecture "Chesterton & Autism," delivered at the 2022 Society of G.K. Chesterton Conference in Milwaukee, Wisconsin. The theme of the conference was "Learning to Think Again," which I thought was a perfect slogan for my speech.)

Everybody who knows even a little about the life of G.K. Chesterton knows that he had a brain with remarkable abilities, and he was also known for eccentric and distinctive behaviors. Chesterton had the ability to dictate an essay to his secretary while writing something totally different in longhand, which was critical to his prodigious output. Chesterton had no qualms about criticizing popular opinions and conventions, and he stood out physically as well as intellectually. Chesterton was known for his unique regular wardrobe and was notoriously absent-minded, on one occasion getting on a train, forgetting where he needed to go, and having to telegraph his wife to find out where he was supposed to be (her answer was "home.")

In recent years, several people familiar with Chesterton's life and work have started to wonder if he was autistic. With his behaviors, unconventional characteristics, and intellectual interests, he certainly fits many of the diagnostic criteria for having autism, but as it is hazardous to make a diagnosis based solely on secondary evidence, close to a century after the subject has passed away, the purpose of this talk is not to try to argue that Chesterton was autistic, but to illustrate the critical role that his writings and ideas have had in helping one specific person with autism develop his own mental processes and survive in a world in which it is often quite difficult for the autistic mind to function. As you have probably guessed, that person is me.

I was diagnosed with autism at the age of twenty-eight, and over the years since then, I've done a great deal of research on the subject. If I had been born twenty years later, I would have very likely been diagnosed very early in life. I certainly had many of the classic symptoms, including very intense and focused interests, repetitive behaviors, and heightened response to stimuli. For me, there was one issue that was really difficult for me, and that was connecting with other people, even when I really wanted to interact. Social cues always were and still are a major challenge for me, and my reactions to various situations can be intense and often debilitating. These are classic symptoms of autism.

Before moving further, it is important to ask the question: what is autism? There are a lot of misconceptions about autism out there, and many stereotypes and oversimplifications that muddle the general public's understanding of what autism is and how people with autism deal with the effects of it. Even though autism has been studied for decades, in-depth research into the subject is still a relatively recent avenue of exploration, and there is still a massive amount of information to be learned about it. Much contemporary research requires tearing down the misconceptions that proliferated for a long time. For decades, autism meant severe mental disability that precluded participation in society, but we now know there are different levels of autism. In the past, treatments were shockingly inhumane, with institutionalization, separation from families, and lobotomies being inflicted on autistic people.

Terminology, recommendations for treatment, and diagnostic criteria have evolved dramatically over the years. One general, currently used term is "autism spectrum disorder." This term is hotly debated, as "disorder" is a controversial word for many people. Right now, however, I want to focus on the word "spectrum." It's a very important part of the terminology. There's a saying I really like that goes, "When you've met one person with autism… you've met one person with autism." Autistic people have very diverse personalities, mental processes, and lives, despite being covered by umbrella terminology. Stereotypes about autistic behavior have disseminated exponentially in the wake of broader public awareness. Some people with autism are able to function totally normally in society, while others have serious problems coping with any social situation. Some have severe disabilities, including being nonverbal, and such issues prevent them from holding down a job. Some have intense likes and dislikes toward things that other autistic people are totally neutral towards, and some people with autism can have extreme reactions to certain stimuli.

There are some subcategories of autism, one of which was once referred to as Asperger Syndrome, though that terminology is no longer used in official diagnoses, and has officially been replaced with "autism spectrum disorder." Still, a lot of people continue to use the term Asperger's, as it has a special meaning for them as their first knowledge of a medically recognized reason for why they thought and acted as they did. Additionally, many people object to the term "disorder." I was diagnosed with the Asperger's form of autism, a couple of years before the terminology was changed, but I will continue to use the older terms at times, especially when addressing characteristics that are distinct to this particular form of autism. People with Asperger's are predominately male, though significant numbers of women have been diagnosed, and some researchers believe that the numbers are more or less equal, and the disparity is due to fewer women being diagnosed. Social skills can frequently be a serious challenge for those with Asperger's, and they often have a lot of trouble with nonverbal cues. Many struggle with forming friendships and engaging in social situations, people diagnosed with Asperger's have a much lower probability of forming romantic attachments than the general population. Though each case is unique, some have outstanding memories, high intelligence, cling to routines, and have strong, perhaps even obsessive interests in topics that fascinate them. Nuance, sarcasm, and certain styles of humor may be challenging to understand.

Those are the internal problems that autistic people can face. Unfortunately, some of the biggest challenges people with autism can face are external, coming from other people with an incomplete understanding of how autism works. The reactions people with autism have to various stimuli are not treatable in the same way one can treat a phobia. The reactions autistic people develop in response to anything from sounds to colors to smells are not necessarily based on fear, and repeated exposure can intensify rather than decrease reactions, though this is not always the case, and indeed, some situations, such as social interactions, can be improved with familiarity. The important point is that autistic reactions must not be labelled with neuroses.

Another problem is the minimizing of this condition. It's quite common to hear comments such as "Oh, you're just shy." Or "You need to get over it. Lots of people are uncomfortable in social situations." Or, "Stop being so inflexible." Or, "Stop talking about that. You're being weird." Or, "Don't you realize you're being annoying?" The fact is, autism is much more than a little awkwardness or an attachment to a routine or a narrow highly focused interest. It's a distinct wiring of the brain, a way of thinking, reacting, and feeling that is genuinely and markedly different from the vast majority of society, and the complexity of the autistic experience is something that is very hard to convey to people who do not personally experience it.

One analogous condition I use from time to time is dyslexia. People understand that a dyslexic brain is wired to process information differently from the vast majority of people, causing them to process images, letters, and words differently. Some dyslexic people may look at a page of text and see letters backwards or upside-down compared to how most people see them, or perhaps they see the words move or spin around on the page. I repeat, autism is a spectrum, so the descriptions of my experiences may only be partly similar to those of other people, or may even be quite different from others. Just like there's a "Type One" and "Type Two" diabetes, people with autism have started to be categorized with differently numbered or lettered types of autism, as reactions can be so radically dissimilar, and I suspect that in the decades to come, classification will become more nuanced and specific.

Autism is <u>not</u> a form of mental illness, and it cannot be "cured," and indeed, many people with autism take umbrage to the fact that it is often thought of as a disease. Some experts estimate that a little under one percent of children fall somewhere on the autism spectrum. Some cases can be very mild, others are debilitating. Some doctors contend that people with certain forms of autism cannot enjoy a high quality of life. In Canada, some circles advocate that autism should be considered grounds for euthanasia along with mental illness in general, a position that has caused a sharp backlash from autism and mental health advocates.

The number of children diagnosed with autism has risen dramatically in recent years, though this is most likely not due to some force causing more autism, but to heightened awareness of what autism is and how to identify it.

I often find myself wondering what my life would have been like if I'd been diagnosed as a child. Today, kids with autism get personalized counseling. I was lucky, I grew up in a loving and supportive family with parents trained in psychology and psychiatry, but it wasn't until I reached adulthood that the diagnostic criteria were better refined. The concept of the autism spectrum, where people could be high-functioning in many respects while still being disabled in other ways by autism, was not widely understood. For a long time, autism diagnoses were only applied to people with a particularly severe form. It's only been about two decades since a substantially revised and more thorough understanding of autism has made its way throughout the psychiatric and psychological disciplines. There's been a lot of debate in mental health circles over how to define whether or not someone has autism, and two different doctors may disagree on whether to diagnose someone as autistic or not. I am sure that in the decades to come, the diagnostic criteria will continue to change. But increasingly, I do not believe that an effective understanding of autism can come solely through the analysis of psychologists and psychiatrists, but by the input of people with autism themselves, as no one knows the workings of their minds better than they do. Still, it can be a severe challenge to explain what's going on in your head, especially when you're not sure of a baseline of how the average person thinks. I know it took me a very long time to be able to put my own experiences into words, and it's a great challenge to do so, because delving into old memories brings back a cascade of old emotions and reactions, but in order to clarify what autism is, I need to delve into my life story, and the role that Chesterton played in helping me.

Growing up, attending the University School of Milwaukee, I frequently felt it impossible to connect to my peers, and social situations were often torturous for me. Without formal training to assist me, I had to help myself find my own pathway to functioning better socially, and I found it through the venue that was most comfortable for me: books.

There are three authors who have been absolutely critical to my mental development process, and I discovered all of them between the ages of eight and twelve. The first was Sir Arthur Conan Doyle, whose Sherlock Holmes stories were pivotal to my observation and deduction skills. Sherlock Holmes taught me how the world could be seen and understood rather than just experienced. The second was Agatha Christie. I read all of her mystery novels between the ages of ten and twelve, and they were crucial not only in refining my logical thinking skills, but also helping me understand why people behaved as they did. The concept of lying or hiding one's true thoughts and goals, was confusing to me, and figuring out the identity of murderers through fair play detective stories helped me understand how people can try to deceive you, and how you can figure out when someone's not being truthful. And the third, of course, was Chesterton. After finishing all of Christie's books, I started looking for new mysteries to read, and after being underwhelmed by most contemporary writers, I started looking for more authors from the Golden Age of Mystery, noted that Chesterton was occasionally referenced in Christie's books, and soon, I found a complete volume of the Father Brown mysteries and read it over spring break of seventh grade.

The Secret of Father Brown is famous for describing the priest's tactics for placing himself in the minds of the criminals he pursues. His "secret" is his ability to replicate the psychology and the souls of perpetrators. He observes actions and determines what mentality is needed to create such a mindset, and he thinks as hard as he can until he believes that he has created an exact copy of the mental workings of the criminal he seeks to identify. This was a revelation for me, and I decided to try it, though not to solve crimes, just the mystery of how to figure out why other people act as they do. Everyone I met, whether it was a teacher, a friendly classmate, a bully, or even the grumpy lunch lady, I tried to explore their minds based on what I knew about them. I worked hard during my spare time to analyze a person and really think about what made that person who they were. I can't claim to have perfectly replicated their minds, and in most cases, the image of them that I created probably bore no connection to the real person, but after following the lead of Father Brown, suddenly, the people at school ceased being impenetrable enigmas and I think that's how I started forming real friendships.

One of the most pernicious and damaging misconceptions about people with autism is that they have no capacity for empathy. This is a monstrous slur. The vast majority of autistic people are very capable of feeling empathy, and many exhibit extremely intense compassion towards people they care about – but there is an important issue that has been misconstrued. Not all, but many people with certain forms of autism can have far more difficulty *understanding the thoughts and motivations of people whose mindsets, opinions, and reactions differ from theirs*. It is a critical distinction. What is often unfairly mistaken for lack of empathy is actually a heightened challenge in comprehending other thought and emotion processes. It is not that we do not *care*, it is that we do not *understand*, and that's a massive difference.

The more I trained myself through reading Chesterton (as well as Doyle and Christie), the more I was able to connect.

It was not just improved relationships with my peers, it was academic success as well.

    I need to stress that the effects of autism on the human mind are not entirely negative. On the contrary, people with autism, due to looking at situations from different ways, can bring innovation and creativity to many fields, as they can think outside a metaphorical box that constrains people used to following more conventional lines of thought. Reading the mysteries of Chesterton and Christie and Doyle helped enhance my mental abilities. Looking at the Father Brown mysteries, or the whodunits of Agatha Christie, or the observational powers of Sherlock Holmes, all helped me learn close attention to detail, or how to break free of arbitrary intellectual constrictions, or that the obvious is not always true. The fantasy writer Neil Gaiman recently wrote about how many Chinese educators were disappointed in how their students lacked the capacity to produce original thought. They could follow instructions and memorize facts, but they could not be innovative. Another commentator (not from Gaiman's essay) observed that one business teacher in China noticed that if he gave an example about starting a business and used a fast-food restaurant as an example, all of the students would write about fast-food restaurants for their projects. Returning to Gaiman, he wrote that in an effort to figure out how to improve their students' abilities, the researchers questioned as many of the most creative and innovative American minds as they could, and found that to a person, all of them had extensively read fantasy books when they were young. This led to the theory that creativity came from thinking about not just what exists, but what could exist with the power of imagination. And a person's future mental trajectory is dependent upon one's reading material and mental exercises from childhood. I really believe that just as fantasy may lead to enhanced creativity, reading fair play mysteries that depend upon logic, observation, and lateral thinking can shape one's mental abilities as well. By the way, I should mention that I read a lot of fantasy growing up, as well.

But no matter how much you try to shape your mind, there's only so much you can do. You can build up your brainpower just like you can build your muscles, but you can't repair an injury through sheer force of will. And when your brain is wired a certain way to provide a response to a stimulus, it often cannot be reprogrammed.

Please try an experiment. Take your right leg, stick it out, and start drawing a clockwise circle with your big toe. Keep going, keep rotating your foot over and over, and do not stop. Now stick out your right hand and keep your eye on your foot. Quickly, draw a circle in the air with your right index finger, but do it *counter*-clockwise. Did you see what happened? Try it again. You will notice that even though your brain sent signals to your foot to keep turning clockwise, when your finger started turning counter-clockwise, your foot automatically turned counter-clockwise as well, even though you did not try to change its direction.

I use this as an example of how our brains are wired. We try to behave in a certain manner, and we may think we're in control of ourselves, such as our movements, but then there's a little stimulus that sends everything going in a totally different direction. Just as turning your right index finger counter-clockwise will reverse the clockwise rotation of your right foot, dozens, even hundreds of stimuli can affect the brain of an autistic person. A certain sound, the wrong smell, the sight of something unpleasant, even the wrong texture can trigger a flood of memories or a reaction that can paralyze me physically or mentally. Unlike most people, I cannot take an argument. When someone starts yelling at me, I start flashing back to scores of previous arguments, and I start feeling intense stabbing pains from my head to my toes. I cannot respond, I cannot think, all I can do is react. Often I become violently ill soon afterwards.

Though following Father Brown's advice really helped me connect with my peers better, and led to more and deeper friendships than I'd ever had previously, just because Chesterton had helped train me to understand (or at least *think* I understood people better and how to more effectively interact around them), that didn't mean that social situations were much easier or fun for me. As everyone who's ever been to high school knows, they are busy places. When you're constantly surrounded by people, bombarded with constant noises, lots of smells, and the unyielding stress that comes from a rigorous curriculum, it's easy to be overwhelmed.

I need to explain the phenomenon of what I call an "Asperger's moment." It's a sudden, intense burst of sensory experience that temporarily leaves me unable to function properly, or even move or speak. It's comparable to a panic attack, but the two reactions are very different, as I know from having battled both. In a panic attack, I can freeze up, feeling my pulse race, my muscles tighten, especially in my chest, and my brain stops working. I can't think, and my mind is largely blank aside from feelings of pain and danger.

An "Asperger's Moment" is comparable, but its nature is quite different. An "Asperger's Moment" is triggered by a memory or a sensory trigger, and instead of my mind freezing up, my brain runs rampant. Uncontrollable visual images flash through my mind, I hear countless sounds, and I pick up numerous smells, tastes, and textures as well. It is literally a case of too much information. I often start shaking, and my hands get clammy. Other than temporary paralysis, the only main point of comparison between panic attacks and Asperger's moments is a racing pulse. Both require a recovery period of at least a few hours, and often I don't fully recuperate from either experience until after a full night of sleep.

Throughout middle and high school, the constant barrage of noise and other people led to multiple Asperger's moments every day, causing me to rush to the bathroom just in time to be sick. The most worrying aspect of all of this was dreading that the wrong person would come in leaving me to be branded with an unflattering nickname that would haunt me for the rest of my life. I rarely socialized with my friends on the weekends, as after five days of being surrounded by people, I needed to be alone with my family for a couple of days to recuperate. Whenever I had a free period junior or senior year, I would retreat to the quietest and emptiest parts of the school I could find, usually corners of the library reading room, and silently do homework or read to recuperate so I had the strength to face the rest of the day.

In my attempt to recreate my experiences, I have to reiterate that my autistic reactions are not always negative. Autistic brain wiring has helped me academically and professionally in countless ways, because I can remember lots of details in narratives, follow logical mathematical principles, and pursue topics of interest to me. I have a very strong memory when it comes to personal experiences and things that interest me. In contrast, it is very challenging for me to remember details that I cannot fit into a clearly flowing narrative, and distractions can hurt me when I'm trying to take a test. But when I enjoy something, I really enjoy it. I develop strong attachments towards people and things I like, and high school started out rough for me, but the more I used the principles of Father Brown to try to understand people better, I started deriving more emotional support from friends. It took a long time, but by my junior year my connection to the University School of Milwaukee – or USM – had grown so strong that my school, along with my home, are the only two places in the world where I've ever felt really happy and comfortable.

But the downside with finally feeling like you belong someplace is that eventually you're forced to leave. While most of my peers couldn't wait to start afresh at college, I felt that my world was ending. And in many ways, that was true. When I was separated from my family and nearly all of my friends, college was extremely difficult for me. Surrounded by constant dormitory noise and having no respite or place of comfort, I lived for the weekends when I could return home and recover. But it was not just the surroundings that affected me, it was my studies as well. You hear a lot today about people wanting to see people who "look like them" in their entertainment. I had a comparable problem. I was reading so many books by the world's leading minds in all sorts of topics, and I found that I had yet to find a single person who I felt *thought* like me.

It was not until midway through my sophomore year of college that, at the end of one exhausting day, I decided to take a break by using the fairly new invention of a search engine to look up some favorite authors, wondering what I'd find. Eventually, I decided to type in Chesterton, and it led me straight to what was then the American Chesterton Society and *Gilbert!* magazine. Before then, I had not read anything of Chesterton other than mystery stories.

I had been largely underwhelmed with many of the famous names we'd been assigned to read in college, but Chesterton was different. I started reading every Chesterton essay I could find, following the way he made an argument, the ways he drew upon all sorts of references to enhance the verbal portraits he was creating, and, after being disappointed by acclaimed novel after acclaimed novel that I found flat and soulless, I started developing my theories that there had to be a better way to write literature, create characters, and shape narratives, all inspired by Chestertonian perspectives.

But there was more than that. After reading Chesterton's *Manalive*, I learned that behaving and thinking differently from other people wasn't necessarily wrong, especially when their ingrained mental habits are making them miserable. Sometimes it takes someone with a different kind of mind to see alternatives or see the nonsensical in the conventional. Autistic people are continually frustrated by people whose opinions are very different from their own.

The Ball and the Cross showed me how even when you fiercely disagree with someone, you can find a way to argue with respect, and recognize the decency and honor in that person.

I don't want to go into every single detail, but college was not much fun for me until I found Chesterton. Afterwards, following his influence, learning seemed more beneficial and even thrilling again. I eventually earned *magna cum laude* on a literary honors project inspired by Chesterton, and right after graduation I presented at my first Chesterton conference.

The next two years were largely positive ones for me. I returned home to Milwaukee and started my master's degree in history from Marquette. With my brain's focus on narratives and the effects of actions and their consequences, concentrating entirely on history meant that my classes were invigorating, even exhilarating from me. For the most part, aside from the crowded bus rides to and from school, I was doing well until April 30th 2006, just a couple of weeks before wrapping up my degree, when my mind shattered. I had the first of a series of migraines, the most powerful and crippling pain I ever felt in my life. For nearly a month, hardly a day went by when I was not laid low by the feeling that a white-hot poker was battering me around the head. I do not know if it was lasting damage from the migraines themselves, or the medications I was taking to stop the pain, or a combination of the two, but when the worst of the migraines subsided in the middle of June, my mind was not what it was just two months earlier. For all my life, I wondered what it would be like to live without all of the reactions that I now know to be part of the autistic experience. After the migraines, I did not feel the same strong reactions to stimuli like smells and sounds, and I did not freak out the same way after being touched by a stranger, and my mind did not start racing at any moment, and I did not flash back to fifty memories at the slightest trigger. In fact, I lost access to many of my memories. But it was not a relief. I did not feel much of anything at all.

For years, my brain felt sluggish and in a perpetual fog. Where once I could not type fast enough to write down all of my ideas for essays, it became a continual challenge to string together enough words to make a single sentence. On a really bad day, it was enough of an uphill battle to arrange enough letters to make actual words. Where once my memory could hold thousands of books and full-sensory memories of the lion's share of my life, now my memories were disjointed and incomplete, and I routinely came to the end of a page without any memory of what I had just read. I found myself digging through old photographs and yearbooks, desperate to find something that would help me piece together a broken memory. All of my assignments took at least four times as long as they once did, leaving me with hardly any time for anything fun. I do not know how I managed to battle my way through ten more classes and work as a teacher's assistant as well, but I flunked my first round on doctoral qualifying exams and had to devote all my efforts to studying for another six months before I managed to pass my second attempt. Incidentally, it was right after I failed my first round of DQEs that I was diagnosed with Asperger's.

There was one exercise that helped me– my work as a columnist for the magazine *Gilbert!* By that point, I was writing reviews of books, movies, and television shows, and before working, I routinely read or reread some of Chesterton's literary criticism for inspiration. I don't know exactly how to explain it, but I think that served as the background for helping me to teach myself to think again. Chesterton always delved into the heart of what an author said, or the complex nature of a person's arguments, and by applying this kind of critical lens to a creative work, I felt as though I could feel my mind getting stronger again.

But I was still in rough shape, and I started going to mass at least once a week, sometimes more, when I was at Marquette. For most of my life, whenever I've been inside a Catholic church, I've had what I now realized were Asperger's reactions due to hyperstimuli. I never got this in churches of other denominations, incidentally. Make of that what you will. But I could attend mass without feeling sick or overwhelmed.

Unfortunately, my mind still wasn't right. In early 2012, nearly six years after the migraines hit and after nearly four years of working on my dissertation, I had nothing usable. I had tons of notes and absolute garbage in terms of written work. Seriously, looking over my dissertation work from 2009 to the start of 2012, I am appalled. It was, quite simply, awful prose with no insight whatsoever into the subject. I could barely turn out a paragraph a day, and with the seven-year deadline from the start of beginning the Ph.D. program looming in just over thirteen months, I was faced with the very real possibility that I might not get my degree.

Then the miracle happened. From the time I graduated from USM, it was my dream job to come back and teach there. In mid-March of 2012, I saw a job opening for a U.S. history teacher job, and I applied for it that night. For a month, I spent most of the day dreaming how I would teach if I got the job, and I would lie in bed, unable to sleep, wondering how I'd handle all of the challenges of the position. I cannot explain it, but that's when my brain started coming alive again. This was the first time since the migraines hit that I genuinely felt that my best days could be ahead, not behind me. And this hopeful, optimistic possibility started to reawaken the imagination and excitement that had lain dormant for nearly six years. Memories I thought were lost forever came flooding back. For years, I had much more trouble with puzzles like the Jumble in the newspaper, but for the first time in six years, I was able to use my imagination and feel actual happiness on a daily basis.

After one month of this, I was not completely better, but I was sharper than I'd been in over half a decade. Long-lost memories came flooding back, and my short-term memory was exponentially stronger. My writing had improved dramatically. And then I got the crushing news that I had not gotten the job. I was devastated. For a few hours I started spiraling downwards, and then something pulled me back up – the knowledge that long after I'd given up hope of being able to think and imagine the way I used to, I was doing better. After years of never being more than fifty or sixty percent, much less on a bad day, I was now around seventy-five percent.

I had stopped reading much for fun, as I couldn't remember new books. Then, seeking comfort, I picked up old favorites, like the Father Brown mysteries and Agatha Christie novels, and rereading them started to open the floodgates. Marcel Proust was famous for writing about all the memories that come back when eating a madeleine. I received comparable reactions with eating all sorts of foods, wearing certain clothing, seeing sights, hearing music, and other everyday actions. Memories I thought were lost forever would come back after hearing a few notes from a 1990's song on the television, or eating a food I hadn't had in years, or pulling on an old jacket.

When I reread Chesterton's "The Invisible Man," I remembered the lessons I learned about how most people overlook obvious details because they don't fit in the bend of their minds. "The Chief Mourner of Marne" reminded me how much more there can be to a story than what people think they know. And the healing continued. The positive and the negative came back. My dissertation writing got exponentially better, and I could turn out five, even ten strong pages a day. I could remember evidence without sifting for hours through my notes to find the little details I needed. But for the first time in six years, the Asperger's moments were coming back. I was shaking, I was getting overwhelmed with floods of memories, and most of all, I was getting terrible reactions at mass again. A few months earlier I could sit in a pew without feeling overstimulated. Now, nearly every time I attended, I broke out into cold sweats, and I had to rush out right afterwards, or even before mass ended, and once again, I became violently ill – or close to it.

After successfully getting my Ph.D. (as well as an additional Masters of Library and Information Science two years later) I noticed that not only had my mental abilities – both helpful and debilitating – gotten stronger than ever, but I had challenges I needed to address. When I turned thirty-three, I decided I needed to officially enter the Catholic Church, having spent most of my adulthood having my religious views formed by Chesterton, but I had a problem, as my reactions at mass were growing much stronger, leading me to feel dizzy in the middle of most services. Thankfully, Fr. Jacob Strand, then at St. Monica's in Whitefish Bay, had some training in working with autistic people, and he helped me through a unique preparation program. I have been watching televised masses and attending mass at a small chapel in a retirement home, and this allows for less powerful reactions, most of the time, though I still get tremors and nausea just watching mass on television. I found myself making steady progress in handling social situations, which had started getting stickier since I began recovering from the migraines, and I started doing exponentially better in 2018 when I got a job as a substitute teacher at USM. Since the pandemic began, however, my autistic reactions have gotten much stronger, matching the intensity I felt at their high point during puberty. A lot of this has to do with having much less social contact, making the rarer interactions more intense, as well as the added pressures coming with social situations now. Travelling has always been a challenge for me, and lately I've had to battle strong Asperger's moments just riding in a car or being in a room with more than a couple of people in it. Being unable to see people's faces through masks hurts my interaction, and having trouble breathing through a mask is a problem too, as I tend to breathe improperly when I'm agitated, such as when I'm in a crowded social situation.

    So now that I've traced the development of my thinking process, I need to explain some more details of it, particularly how I see the world. I don't just see the present. I see the past and the potential future as well. If any of you are familiar with the classic television series *Upstairs, Downstairs*, the iconic closing scene (if you will please excuse some very minor spoilers) is comparable to my own experiences. This will not provide much in the way of spoilers for those of you who have not seen the series, but in the show's last few minutes, Rose, the longtime servant, walks through the empty rooms of the house where she has worked for a quarter century. As she moves around, she hears snippets of conversations she has had over the years, as the memories come flooding back. The difference between Rose's nostalgia and my own experiences is that I do not just hear dialogue from the past. I actually see images from the past as well, not as clearly as they appear in real life, but faintly, almost ghostlike. It can make it very hard to talk to someone when one is trying to talk over multiple conversations one has had with the same person in the same place. If I look at someone I've known for a while, I do not just see them as they are now. I can see their clothing and hairstyle and other appearance changes from how I've seen them over the years, flashing back in forth in front of me.

In recent years, adaptors of Sherlock Holmes have toyed with the ideas that Holmes may have a form of autism, though no official diagnosis has ever been made in any production. Nevertheless, they've managed to replicate my own mind workings, and those of many other autistic people. In the Robert Downey Jr. movies, Holmes routinely plans out every action he takes before he does it, anticipating consequences and the steps he needs to take to achieve the outcome he wants. When I first saw this, I was stunned, as it was an uncanny recreation of my own mental processes. Comparably, in the Benedict Cumberbatch television series *Sherlock*, Holmes's observations about people and objects come in the form of little word descriptions that can be seen hovering around the relevant object, which is a mental reaction I often have when I'm trying to visually process my surroundings.

Of the many challenges that come with autism, one of the harshest is the difficult nature of explaining how our minds work and the nature of their reactions. If I try to explain why I feel angry, I don't just feel emotions about what made me angry recently, I mentally relive dozens of incidents where I felt similar anger simultaneously, and I become overloaded with emotion and unable to express my thoughts.

One of the biggest stumbling blocks to a fuller understanding of autism and helping people who have it with related challenges is the fact that autistic people's personal perspectives on their neurological state have been overshadowed in the professional sphere by doctors who have compressed, oversimplified, and distorted the autistic experience in order to fit neat diagnostic categories. In the public sphere, writers and dramatists of varying capability have handles portrayals of autism to mixed results. Some authors have done brilliant work in capturing the complexity of autism and presenting it in an unconventional but effective manner to the general public. Maybe the most popular and successful creative work to try to convey the autistic mindset to the general public is Mark Haddon's novel *The Curious Incident of the Dog in the Night-Time*, and its award-winning stage play adaptation. In this story, Christopher John Francis Boone, a teenager who clearly has a form of autism, but as in many presentations of such minds in books and entertainment, he is not given an official diagnosis, as people seem distinctly reluctant to put official names to these kinds of mental workings. After reading the book, which depicts the character trying to solve the mystery of the death of his neighbor's dog, I felt as if Christopher Boone's voice were exactly the same as my own mental workings when I was fifteen. His interests and reactions mirrored my own so closely, that aside from the very different perspectives toward religion between us, it felt like Haddon was looking into my mind when he wrote the book. The stage version has used numerous lighting and special effects to mimic Christopher Boone's mental workings, and though not all of them really reflect how I personally think and react, they serve as useful ways to make intangible experiences visible. In the past decade or so, there has been an explosion of artistic depictions of autism in film and television, especially in the mystery genre, of varying quality and depth. Others have reduced autism to a one- or two-dimensional set of quirks and affectations that dilute autism to mere difficult behavior and general "weirdness" in the eyes of others.

Despite an improved understanding of autism proving to be a critical aid to many people on the spectrum, with familiarity has come new misconceptions and challenges. Some people who have never been officially diagnosed like to declare that they identify as autistic, trumpeting their condition in a way that has been derisively referred to as "autism chic." In contrast, increased awareness has not brought universal understanding. If there is one misrepresentation of autism that really upsets me, it's the use of the pejorative phrase "sperging out" when someone starts ranting or freaking out or rambling about a topic solely of interest to them. There's a widespread belief in many circles that autism is not actually real, and it's just a trendy excuse for neuroticism. I hope that by talking about these issues as I'm doing now, I can help to dispel these misconceptions.

This lecture was by far the most difficult thing I've ever had to write in my life. I've been working on this for months, and it's been an uphill battle to get more than a few sentences put on paper at a time. I suppose this is because it's so personal, and because it's so difficult to describe the autistic experience. Over the past couple of years, I've started a very disorganized outreach program for people connected to the Milwaukee Archdiocese for people with autism and the people who love them. Many autistic people have severe reactions at church, and it leads many of them to leave and never come back. This is a big issue that is only starting to be addressed.

A lot of people with autism need help, especially children who don't realize that most other people see the world differently from them. They need guidance with their education and personal relationships, and later they need help with the job market. Today, many young people get help throughout their formal schooling, but then when they graduate, they lose a lot of their support, and the results can leave them adrift and feeling helpless.

Many people think that the way to help autistic people is to train them to act and behave like neurotypical people, but based on personal experience, I find that is often not a feasible goal, and that autism is not meant to be erased but assisted. Conformity with general society should be supplanted with accommodation and understanding.

I do not see myself as a victim, just as someone who thinks and responds differently from most people. I am, however, very concerned about autistic people who have it worse than I do and cannot explain or protect or take care of themselves, and do not have caring families or support systems.

In "The Eye of Apollo," there is the idea that any ailment can be cured if the mind is quite steady. Father Brown knew this to be a lie, and I know that the many people who firmly believe that autistic people need to be chastised or browbeaten into what is seen as acceptable behavior are perpetuating this falsehood.

I still have a lot of problems that I'm trying to overcome that are connected to the way that my mind works. Like many autistic people, I have trouble finding full-time work, though I have multiple part-time jobs that allow me to work at home, and my dating experiences have been singularly awkward and unsuccessful. But I am not giving up – not by a long shot.

I do not know if Chesterton had a form of autism himself, but whether he did or not, he and his work and life stand as an inspiration for me to keep going and never surrender to despair. I did not have the guidance many autistic children have today, but Chesterton was one of the formative influences who helped me survive and thrive, and for that, I will be eternally grateful.

CHAPTER TWO
A Collection of Potentially Autistic Fictional Sleuths

(WARNING: As this is an analysis of numerous mystery series, spoilers will be found throughout the book. I will try to minimize them wherever possible, but please read with caution.)

Over the decades, hundreds of popular fictional detectives on film and television have entertained viewers. With very few exceptions, these detectives are intelligent, observant, and likeable characters. Lieutenant Columbo, Jim Rockford, Jessica Fletcher, Lennie Briscoe, Jane Tennison, Joe Friday, Joe Mannix, and countless others have earned massive fan bases, and their series continue to be popular viewing, even decades after their last episodes aired. Most successful television detectives are distinctive characters played by charismatic actors, and there's no set formula for creating an iconic sleuth. The detective may be an official member of law enforcement, a private investigator, or a total amateur. The character may be the product of a successful book series, or an entirely original creation. No background, ethnicity, personal beliefs, or approach is prohibitory to success.

Many detectives have also dealt with significant personal challenges, such as illnesses and disabilities. Robert T. Ironside used a wheelchair after being shot. Andy Sipowicz battled alcoholism for eleven seasons on *NYPD Blue*. On *Cracker*, Edward "Fitz" Fitzgerald struggled with smoking, drinking, and gambling addictions. But in the twenty-first century, a new trend emerged, as an increasing number of television and movie detectives exhibited characteristics that arguably placed them on the autism spectrum. This coincides with a general explosion in characters with autism in the media, not just in crime shows, but in dramas and comedies, crafted with varying degrees of skill and sensitivity. I am focusing on the phenomenon of the autistic sleuth because these portrayals tend to express how certain mental functions can be both useful and challenging for the autistic.

Before continuing, it is as essential that I clarify the purpose of this list, especially since only a tiny minority of the detectives are explicitly diagnosed with autism. In many cases, some psychologists or psychiatrists might disagree on whether or not the characters in question qualify. This chapter is *not* trying to argue that all of these characters have autism. The critical point being made here is that *they exhibit qualities that real-life people with autism may be able to use in order to illustrate their own mental processes, personal difficulties, and other issues that they may have trouble conveying through words.* Incomplete understandings and misconceptions about autism stem from the difficulty of finding words sufficiently adequate to replicate the autistic experience. Personally, I and other people I know with autism have found that using depictions of characters– even if they may not definitively have autism – can be valuable tools in conveying their social and mental challenges to others.

Once again, autism is a spectrum, and it is critical to understand that just because a character has autism, that does not mean that all autistic people share those reactions and thought patterns. I am in no way trying to suggest that the characteristics of autism depicted in the productions shown here are more common than others, nor am I trying to minimize alternative forms of autism. However, the portrayals illustrated here, in general, more closely match my own experiences; hence, I am more comfortable analyzing them. The fact that I have decided to focus on crime shows is admittedly based in part on my own obsession with mysteries, and for the sake of a manageable focus. I'm a fan of most of the shows and movies discussed here, though in a couple of cases, a character from a work I don't particularly enjoy has been included for the sake of completeness. I hope that my lack of enthusiasm in a couple of cases isn't obvious, though in most instances I think my affection for the franchise is evident. Additionally, I am aware of the numerous non-mystery shows that prominently feature autistic characters, from *Atypical* to *Parenthood* to *Sesame Street*. These are excluded in order to limit the scope to a manageable amount. This isn't meant to a comprehensive overview of all portrayals of autism in the media. But by portraying autistic people as sleuths, these productions place particular focus on the way the characters' minds work, and I think that covering this niche is particularly useful for analytical purposes.

    I want to make it unequivocally clear that in many cases, where an official diagnosis has not been made on-screen, ambiguity and controversy are bound to occur. Many of these characteristics, such as anxiety, social awkwardness, and interest in specialized subjects are in no way limited to people with autism. A neurotypical person's mind may have many points of similarity with an autistic brain. When diagnosing autism, it's often a considerable number of combined factors that lead to the sum total of a diagnosis, and there are many individuals who fall into a borderline category, where one well-trained professional might confidently state that an individual has autism (perhaps using the controversial term "high-functioning"), another equally respected mental health expert could be adamant that the same person does not exhibit sufficient characteristics to qualify as autistic. Additionally, on any given day, a "fringe" autistic individual may or may not appear reasonably neurotypical due to various factors. I know from personal experience that my publicly discernable autistic characteristics can be heightened or subdued due to numerous influences, like the amount of sleep that I get.

Furthermore, it's critical to note that an actor portraying a character will often present traits very differently from real-life people. Actors play roles and sometimes put particular emphasis (or less politely, ham up) certain qualities at the expense of verisimilitude, and screenwriters are just as susceptible to believing that they can make their art more interesting, entertaining, and dramatic, than real life. It should also be noted that the long-running police procedurals discussed on this show often have large writers' rooms with heavy turnover over the years. With so many cooks in the kitchen, and varying creative visions, knowledge of characters, and decisions to "evolve" the character, it is common for there to be inconsistencies or the occasional action that might seem out of character.

Throughout this chapter, I am going to address the history of potentially autistic detectives roughly chronologically, but with a certain degree of flexibility for comparative issues. I will begin by addressing recent reinterpretations of arguably the most famous fictional detective of them all: Sherlock Holmes, who first appeared in print in 1887.

For more than a century and a quarter, readers have wondered how the mind of Sherlock Holmes works. Actors and screenwriters have all brought their own interpretations of what formed the Great Detective's brain over the decades. Many prominent portrayers, such as Basil Rathbone, never delved too deeply into the depths of Holmes' psyche, preferring instead to focus on his investigations and triumphs, portraying Holmes as both a thinking man's thinking man and also a man of action, with no attempt to place a label upon the brain beneath the deerstalker.

But as the twentieth century progressed, creatives became increasingly interested in diagnosing Holmes. Nicholas Meyer created a formative event in Holmes' youth in his 1974 novel *The Seven-Per-Cent Solution* and the subsequent film adaptation. In that story, Sigmund Freud extracts a long-suppressed memory from Holmes' mind, where Holmes' mother had an affair, leading to Holmes' father killing his adulterous wife before committing suicide, and the trauma eventually shaped Holmes' passion for catching wrongdoers and led to his eventual self-medicating with cocaine. In contrast, Billy Wilder initially planned to portray Holmes as a repressed or even unconsciously gay man in his 1970 film *The Private Life of Sherlock Holmes*, causing a powerful impact on the character's personal life. In the final version of the film, this portrayal was changed to unconfirmed implications and subtext. Jeremy Brett, who played Holmes in a decade-long series of television adaptations, battled bipolar disorder, and occasionally suggested in his performances that Holmes had a similar mental illness. A BBC radio series starring Clive Merrison as Holmes had Watson expressly theorize in one episode that Holmes had manic depressive tendencies. As the twentieth century ended, a new potential diagnosis frequently came to be directed towards Holmes – autism.

It must be reiterated that this chapter is not trying to argue that the Sherlock Holmes of Conan Doyle's stories was definitely autistic. Certainly there was no scientific understanding of the condition at the time that they were written, and not all of Holmes' distinctive character traits discussed here are necessarily unique to autism. The point is to illustrate that it *could be theorized* that Holmes demonstrates certain autistic characteristics.

There are certainly numerous passages in the original Canon that can – and do – inspire today's readers to suggest an autism diagnosis for Holmes. Early in the first Holmes novel, *A Study in Scarlet*, Watson is nonplussed by his new roommate's frankness, unconventional behaviors, obsession with certain topics, and complete lack of awareness of certain points of common knowledge. It should also be noted that in the four short stories that are narrated in whole or in part by Holmes himself, very little of what he writes reveals any strikingly autistic behaviors or thought patterns. It's only through Watson's eyes that the reader observes Holmes's bluntness, even rudeness, his lack of interest in romantic relationships or friendships, and other eccentricities that put off or perplex other people. Holmes has told Watson that accounts of his cases ought to focus primarily on the problem being solved, with the dramatic and human elements minimized, so it's possible that Holmes' stylistic beliefs (and possibly an unwillingness to share too much personal information) cause him to keep his own personality out of the narrative as much as possible.

But in recent years, some of the most prominent portrayals of Holmes have strongly, though not definitively, attempted to place him on the autism spectrum. Multiple franchises will be covered here. In the case of the Downey movies, they are set in a time long before autism was identified, so while attributes that contemporary viewers might connect with autism might be integrated into Downey's portrayal, no character would ever be able to provide a name for his behavior that would be officially recognized by the medical establishment. In contrast, the twenty-first century-set *Sherlock* takes place in a time when understanding of neurodiversity is more widespread, and a doctor like John Watson, even if he doesn't specialize in psychiatry or neurology, is aware of autism.

The lack of an official diagnosis for Downey's version makes total sense, Cumberbatch's less so. In both cases, not only has Holmes been given certain distinctly autistic mannerisms, but both have also produced stylistic versions of the workings of Holmes' mind that have become hallmarks of their respective series.

One early scene in the 2009 movie *Sherlock Holmes* strongly reflects how a person with autism might respond in a busy social situation takes place in a crowded restaurant. As Holmes waits for his dining companions, Watson (Jude Law) and his fiancée Mary Morstan (Kelly Reilly), Holmes fidgets in his chair, his eyes darting around the room, registering tiny sights and sounds in the cacophony of diners around him, growing steadily more unsettled until the others finally arrive. Other behaviors and mental processes expressed by Downey's Holmes that will be addressed in-depth later are also useful demonstrative tools for illustrating mental processes.

Similarly, Benedict Cumberbatch's portrayal in the television series *Sherlock* also has many characteristics of someone on the autism spectrum. Shortly after Sherlock makes his first appearance, he announces that he considers himself "a high-functioning sociopath." Many viewers and mental health professionals have taken issue with that description. As a skilled psychologist or psychiatrist would be unlikely to make such a diagnosis, it seems most probable that this is a *self-diagnosis*, and a very misguided one. Based on his personal reactions to people and the way he processes emotions, it's certainly within the bounds of probability that an intelligent man with limited knowledge of psychological diagnostics and no compunction against shocking other people might embrace a label that serves to both isolate and distinguish himself.

About the only direct reference to Sherlock having autism in the series comes in the second episode of the second series, "The Hounds of Baskerville."

JOHN. You do know he's actually pleased you're here? Secretly pleased.
LESTRADE. Is he? That's nice. I suppose he likes having all the same faces back together. It appeals to his...his --
JOHN. Asperger's?

As a twenty-first century doctor, it's not surprising that John Watson might consider this diagnosis, even if he doesn't specialize in mental health. More puzzling is the fact that he's never tried to have Sherlock receive an official diagnosis or at least challenge the sociopathy self-diagnosis, although given Sherlock's notoriously difficult personality, it's in-character to suspect that any efforts would have met with resistance.

Most portrayals of Holmes have traditionally been played without a strong autistic suggestion, and of the recent portrayals, any autistic characteristics in Jonny Lee Miller's Holmes in *Elementary* are far less pronounced and debatable. While some viewers might interpret his personality as autistic, others do not. Henry Cavill's performance in the *Enola Holmes* Netflix movies seems pretty neurotypical. Of the many twenty-first century portrayals of Holmes, only a couple demonstrate autistic mannerisms, such as the Japanese gender-swapped *Miss Sherlock* (2018) with Yûko Takeuchi in the title role, solving crimes in modern-day Japan with a similarly feminized Dr. Wato Tachibana (often referred to as "Wato-san"), though unlike the other two portrayals of Holmes discussed here, stylized versions of her mind processes are minimal. At times, such as when she's trying to crack a passcode, words and images briefly flash on-screen, clearly referencing *Sherlock's* stylistic approach. On occasion, Takeuchi's Sherlock seems to have intense reactions to stimuli. In the first episode, she claims to be distracted by bad fashion, and when she interviews a suspect at a nightclub, she is obviously disconcerted by the noise and flashing lights on the floor below her. Later, when she confronts the killer, who then commences shrieking, Sherlock runs to a corner of the room, curls up in fetal position on the sofa, covers her ears, and winces, clearly so distraught by the noise that she takes her eyes off a potentially dangerous person for a minute, leaving herself vulnerable to attack and giving the culprit a chance to escape. In addition, some autism-presenting personality quirks strongly suggest that Takeuchi's Sherlock is on the spectrum, but no official diagnosis, or even suspicion, is ever voiced.

Another Japanese series from 2016, *IQ 246: The Cases of a Royal Genius*, which draws obvious inspiration from the Sherlock Holmes Canon (and to a lesser extent, the character of L from *Death Note*), features Sharaku Homonji (Yûji Oda) a brilliant detective of aristocratic lineage. Certain aspects of his behavior are debatably autistic in nature, and even though his eccentricities could be attributed to many other mental factors, Oda's Homonji will be included in this analysis. The 2019 Japanese series *Sherlock: Untold Stories*, stars Dean Fujioka in a modernized Japan-set series set that draws inspiration from English-language series that move Holmes to contemporary times, and there are suggestions that Fujioka's interpretation is also on the spectrum, but as of this writing *Sherlock: Untold Stories* has not yet been given a subtitled release for English-speaking audiences, so it will not be included in this analysis.

Moving on to detectives created strictly for television, the next character to be profiled is one whose position on the spectrum is most questionable. In 2000, William Petersen's Gil

Grissom on *CSI: Crime Scene Investigation* became a widely recognized figure. A Las Vegas-based scientist with a deep interest in entomology, Grissom led a forensics team for the first several seasons, distinguishing himself with his attention to detail, his dedication to his work, and his detailed knowledge of a wide assortment of subjects.

It should be noted that Grissom's characterization varied considerably over the course of the series. Part of this was due to the wide array of writers working on the show and the comparatively large number of appearances his character made. Many aspects of the show, including Grissom himself, grew darker and grittier as the series progressed, and much of the quirkiness that led some viewers to wonder if Grissom was on the spectrum was toned down or practically eliminated in many later episodes.

Not all detectives solve crimes. Some are physicians who diagnose mysterious illnesses. On the UK series *Doc Martin* (2004-2022), Doctor Martin Ellingham (Martin Clunes), often has to investigate the conditions of patients that defy obvious identification. (While Freddie Highmore's Dr. Shaun Murphy on *The Good Doctor* (an Americanization of the South Korean show), is also a doctor with autism, I have chosen not to discuss it here because the investigative nature of his medical work is less prominent than on *Doc Martin*, and the titular character series *House*, which promoted the term "medical mysteries," is more irascible than distinctly autistic.)

Dr. Ellingham began life as a character without obvious autistic tendencies in the film *Saving Grace* and two spinoff telemovies, but when the series took its final form, his personality became brusque to the point of rudeness. His once-stellar medical career was derailed once he became afflicted by a debilitating fear of blood, so he is forced to relocate to the coastal town of Portwenn as the local physician. Throughout the series, he uses his extensive medical knowledge to uncover obscure conditions afflicting his patients, and also learns to deal with the social fallout of his people skills, as he falls in love with a local schoolteacher and makes friendships without making any effort to be sociable. A mental health professional points out that he might have Asperger's in an early season, but no formal diagnosis is ever made, and Dr. Ellingham does not pursue the matter.

Moving back to shows that are unquestionably crime dramas, Dr. Spencer Reid (Matthew Gray Gubler) on *Criminal Minds* (2005-2020) is another example of a highly intelligent character who exhibits many classic autistic tendencies, though the show itself is reluctant to supply an official diagnosis. As the series begins, Reid is still in his twenties, but he has three doctorates in chemistry, engineering, and mathematics, plus additional degrees. His social awkwardness is a defining character trait, as is his predilection for providing far larger quantities of information than his peers prefer to hear. His intelligence is vital to the Behavioral Analysis Unit of the FBI in catching dangerous predators, but he has lasting concerns over his own mental state, as his mother is institutionalized due to schizophrenia.

Following in the turn-of-the-century trend of detectives who might or might not be on the spectrum, depending on one's opinion and the episode being watched, is Detective Robert "Bobby" Goren (Vincent D'Onofrio) of *Law & Order: Criminal Intent* (2001-2011). Due to certain aspects of his characterization that mirror classic autistic tendencies, Goren falls into the "maybe" category in many discussions of potentially autistic fictional characters, with fans and commentators largely split on the diagnosis. Goren works for the New York City Police Department's Major Case Squad, and is a highly effective detective due to his ability to get inside the minds of suspects and criminals, not only in creating profiles of culprits, but also in his talent for determining psychological pressure points, leading criminals to confess, and suspects and witnesses to provide information they'd rather keep secret. Notably, Goren also uses his interrogation tactics to prove characters' innocence often as well. Though his approaches to crime solving are unconventional, he has built a very close relationship with his primary detecting partner, Detective Alexandra Eames (Kathryn Erbe), and Goren enjoys a stellar career until personal issues and revelations disrupt his work over the second half of the series.

The possibility of Goren being autistic is very rarely broached on the show, but one particular episode, S2, E14's "Probability," features Wally Stevens (Mark Linn-Baker), an undiagnosed autistic man with a sympathetic backstory who is suspected of involvement in a series of deaths. Goren builds a bond with Stevens, despite his crimes, and their connection will be analyzed more deeply in the chapter "The Autistic Criminal."

Adrian Monk (Tony Shaloub) on *Monk* (2002-2009) is a case where some viewers wonder if the central character is, if not *mis*diagnosed, at least *incompletely* diagnosed. No one questions that he has obsessive-compulsive disorder. Monk was a high-achieving detective for the San Francisco Police Force until his beloved wife Trudy (Melora Hardin for most of the series) was murdered by a car bomb. The loss of his wife and the failure to catch the criminal had a crushing effect on Monk. He lost his job, and spent some years recovering until he was able to resume work as a private investigator. He was able to function thanks to the help of his assistants, first Sharona Fleming (Bitty Schram, S1 to halfway through S3), and later

Natalie Teeger (Traylor Howard) midway through S3 through S8). Battling hundreds of phobias, ranging from germs to heights to water to milk to wind, and requiring strict routines and cleanliness levels to function, Monk manages to keep solving cases by confronting his fears and leaning on his supportive allies, with his uncanny powers of observation being pivotal to his sleuthing success.

But while Monk's OCD is not questioned, the possibility that Monk also is on the autism spectrum has never been addressed on the show. Potential links between OCD and autism have been studied for years, and there is substantial overlap where people receive diagnoses for both conditions. Given several issues of characterization, it is debatably possible that Monk's diagnosis is incomplete.

Though not a traditional detective, the character of Chloe O'Brian on *24* and its continuation series *24: Live Another Day* (Mary Lynn Rajskub, joined the show in S3 (2004-2010, 2014)), is a computer expert who uses her information analysis skills to battle terrorists and to unravel conspiracies. Her distinctive personality has led many fans to hypothesize about her being on the autism spectrum, and her technological skills are often critical to identifying and defeating villains. In multiple instances, her analysis of data helps to prove suspects' guilt or innocence. Chloe initially has difficulty connecting with her colleagues, though over the course of the series, she steadily becomes a respected and relied-upon member of an oft-changing counterterrorism team.

On the 2005-2017 series *Bones*, the title character, Dr. Temperance "Bones" Brennan (Emily Deschanel) is widely seen as being on the autism spectrum. A forensic anthropologist with numerous degrees in related subjects, her usefulness in crime solving, thanks to her ability to analyze dead bodies, leads to a second career that runs parallel to her work at the Smithsonian. Paired with FBI Special Agent Seeley Booth (David Boreanaz), an investigator with a sharply contrasting personality to hers, the two solve various crimes, and eventually become romantically involved, marry, and have two children together, though not quite in that order. Though the series is inspired by the crime novels and anthropological career of Kathy Reichs, the character and world in Reich's books only have a loose connection to the television show.

Bones is notoriously socially awkward, and has little knowledge of many subjects outside her area of expertise. Early in the series, when characters make a joke, often based on popular culture, her response of "I don't get it" practically becomes a catchphrase. Her behavior, diction, and relationships with others exhibit many autistic characteristics, though she maintains close friendships with the small group of co-workers who form her investigative team at the Smithsonian. As in many long-running procedurals, Bones' characterization changes a lot over the seasons, as she goes from adamantly denying she wants children to being a loving mother, commits to a relationship, and gains a deeper understanding of other people's mindsets. Despite the widespread belief in Bones' autism, an official diagnosis is never explored.

Unlike Benedict Cumberbatch's Sherlock Holmes, Michael C. Hall's Dexter Morgan on *Dexter* (2006-2013, and the revival series *Dexter: New Blood* (2021-2022)) is most likely a sociopath. Like Tony Shaloub's Adrian Monk, it is possible that Dexter's diagnosis is incomplete, and that he may be on the autism spectrum as well. It is easy for viewers to focus on the more violent aspects of Dexter's character, as he is a serial killer, though he justifies his actions by satisfying his homicidal urges through executing other murderers. Severely psychologically scarred after witnessing the gruesome murder of his mother at a very young age, and then being trapped in the gory crime scene for an extended period of time, Dexter was adopted by the police officer Harry Morgan (James Remar), though his stepfather eventually became disturbed by the violent tendencies that emerged as the boy grew older. In the eighth season, it is revealed that seeking help, Harry turned to what might possibly be the worst possible source for help (depending on one's point of view), Dr. Evelyn Vogel (Charlotte Rampling), a self-proclaimed expert in sociopaths who lionizes them, and may have psychopathic tendencies herself. Dr. Vogel encouraged Harry to allow Dexter to vent his homicidal tendencies in what she believed was an ethical manner – by killing criminals who were a danger to society. Harry accepted this diagnosis, and these guidelines became known as "The Code of Harry."

Especially in the earlier seasons, Dexter shows many traits not just of psychopathy, but also of a form of autism, particularly in his interactions with others, and some other autistic people have informed me that they deeply connect with Dexter's often clumsy attempt to mimic other people's behaviors and his fumbling of social cues. The YouTube critic The Vile Eye, in his video "Analyzing Evil: Dexter Morgan," observes that, "If Dexter hadn't been encouraged to fit the role of a psychopathic serial killer, I think we'd be able to label him as someone suffering from schizophrenia, schizo-titled personality disorder, alexithymia, or even autism."

Given his ability to analyze blood spatter, and his research skills in tracking down criminals, Dexter certainly qualifies as a sleuth even if he is not an official police officer, and given his propensity for homicide, he will be a major figure in the chapter "The Autistic Criminal."

Death Note entered the public consciousness from 2003 to 2006, when it became one of the most popular manga series of all times. Its reputation only grew larger in 2006, with the release of an acclaimed anime adaptation, and the first of a trilogy of live-action Japanese movies. A 2015 live-action Japanese television miniseries followed, and a widely lambasted Americanized Netflix movie was released in 2017. A musical adaptation by American creatives was a hit in Japan and South Korea, with one production being filmed in 2015, and in 2023, a staged concert played to sold-out audiences in England, with the possibility of a fully staged London production and a transfer to Broadway in the future.

Death Note centers around Light Yagami, a high-achieving teenager who is frustrated by all the criminals who go unpunished by society. One day, he comes across a magical book, the Death Note, which has the power to kill anybody who writes that person's true name in it, as long as the writer knows what the intended victim's face looks like. Not only that, but within limits, the manner and time of death may be determined by the writer. Light quickly gets to work executing criminals from around the world, and L, a mysterious detective who notoriously never shows his face, is called in to investigate these inexplicable deaths.

Circumstances compel L to break precedent and reveal his identity to a team of Japanese detectives. He's a fairly young man with a host of idiosyncrasies and behavior quirks that have led many fans to theorize that he has autism. In the manga and anime, his hair is always mussed, there are dark circles under his eyes, his spine is always hunched, he sits in a crouched position and in the anime, he always wears the same outfit – a white long-sleeved t-shirt and blue jeans. He rarely wears shoes or socks if he can help it, and despite his slender build, L subsists entirely on sweets with the occasional piece of fruit. Yet despite – or as in many cases discussed here, perhaps *because of* – his many eccentricities, he's a brilliant detective and a skilled tactician, and much of the appeal of *Death Note* comes from the battle of wits between L and Light.

It should be noted that each depiction of L (the anime, where he is voiced by Kappei Yamaguchi for the Japanese version, and dubbed in English by Alessandro Juliani; the Japanese movies (played by Kenichi Matsuyama), the miniseries (Kento Yamazaki), the Netflix movie (Lakeith Stanfield), and a filmed version of the musical (Teppei Koike)) makes significant changes to the character's actions and ultimate fate (in the live-action miniseries, there is little hint of L having autism), and different portrayals will be explored in more depth later on in this book.

Based on the novels by Alexander McCall Smith, *The No. 1 Ladies' Detective Agency* centers around Mma[*] Precious Ramotswe, a self-taught private detective working in Gaborone, Botswana. At the start of the series, she hires Mma Grace Makutsi, to be her secretary. The one-season 2009 television adaptation is largely loyal to the books in spirit, though it rearranges the order of certain events amongst the episodes. Mma Makutsi, played on the show by Anika Noni Rose, is intelligent and efficient, but also self-consciously distinctive in her mannerisms. She is quite proud of her record-setting score on a secretarial test, earning ninety-seven percent. As portrayed by Rose, her speech patterns and movements reflect several autistic traits, and she pays strict attention to rules, showing no compunction against publicly calling out people who violate them. No one ever mentions the word "autism" on the series, and

---

[*] "Mma" is a traditional form of address preceding a name, meant to show respect.

like many of the characters discussed here, her characterization is best described as "autism-*suggestive*."

Over the course of the book and television series, Mma Makutsi starts taking on investigative roles, using her sharp observational skills to gather useful information, and her contributions are often vital to solving cases, such as a series of deaths that occur with alarming regularity at a hospital, and despite some initial trepidation, she soon finds private detection to be an immensely fulfilling job.

One of the most analyzed characters in twenty-first century crime fiction is Lisbeth Salander, the title character of *The Girl with the Dragon Tattoo*. Many people have suggested that she presents classic symptoms of autism, though many others disagree, preferring to suggest PTSD, sociopathy, psychopathy, anti-social behavior disorder, and other diagnoses. As the series makes a point of never giving an official name for her condition (the diagnosis of one corrupt mental health professional (who has a vested interest of convincing the courts that she must be institutionalized) can safely be discarded), all of these suggestions are pure theory, but as the idea of autism spectrum disorder is commonly floated, it must be addressed in this study.

Salander is a young Swedish computer hacker who had an abusive father, a criminal with strong connections to a secret government agency. When she was young, she tried to protect herself and her mother by throwing gasoline on her father and setting him alight. He survived, and his powerful allies protected him, and Salander was confined to a mental hospital for much of her teenage years, where she was placed in restraints and abused. When she was released, she was placed under a guardian's oversight, and though one guardian was a kindly man before his stroke, the replacement guardian raped her before giving her money from her trust account. The constant failures of the justice system to protect her and to shield her abusers led her to distrust the authorities, and as an adult, she works as a researcher, using her hacking skills. Over the course of the series, she joins forces with an investigative journalist, and eventually turns to vigilantism to confront violent criminals, including many from her own past.

To date, three actresses have played Lisbeth Salander in movies, not counting the young actresses who have portrayed the character as a child in flashbacks. Noomi Rapace played the role in Swedish-language adaptations of the original book trilogy by Stieg Larsson (*The Girl with the Dragon Tattoo*, *The Girl Who Played with Fire*, and *The Girl Who Kicked the Hornet's Nest*, all released in 2009), Rooney Mara took on the part in the 2011 English-language adaptation of the first book, and Claire Foy assumed the character in *The Girl in the Spider's Web* (2018), based upon the continuation novel by David Lagercrantz (as such, the discrepancies in continuity will be addressed in later analysis).

Salander's psyche defies easy analysis, but as her character frequently presents traits commonly seen as autistic, her mentality must be addressed here.

Abed Nadir, played by Danny Pudi on the comedy series *Community*, (2009-2015), is a unique case. He is included in this study in part because of his notable critiques on popular culture's turning the autistic sleuth into a trope. Abed uses popular culture to connect with the world in ways he can better understand. In the first episode, his continuous talking about topics of interest to him leads Jeff Winger (Joel McHale), a lawyer who must earn his degree in order to resume his career, to diagnose Abed with Asperger's, though Jeff has no training in psychology. Abed embodies many of the standard characteristics presented by autistic people, though in the pattern discussed here, his condition is never officially confirmed by a qualified, competent mental health professional. In the third season episode, "Regional Holiday Music," (S3E10) he raps to the camera that whether or not he is on the spectrum is "none of your business."

Though *Community* is not a mystery show, the series often parodies various movies and television shows, and in a *Law & Order* parody (S3E17– "Basic Lupine Urology"), Abed assumes the role of a detective alongside his friend Troy Barnes (Donald Glover), and in the riff of David Fincher and other serial killer movies "Basic Intergluteal Numismatics" (S5, E3), when Dean Craig Pelton (Jim Rash) suggests that Abed's "special" mind might be used to catch the culprit., Abed mimics a stereotypical television autistic sleuth, and says, "I see a man... using a social disorder as a procedural device. Wait, wait, wait, I see another man. Mildly autistic super detectives everywhere. Basic cable, broadcast networks. Pain. Painful writing. It hurts." Later in the episode, Abed is shown removing series like *The Bridge* and *Hannibal* from his digital video recorder. On other occasions, Abed is the only character amongst his friend to notice something wrong, or to determine the truth of a situation. *Community* often critiques popular culture, and the case of Abed Nadir will be used to study the potential shortcomings of the entertainment industry portraying the autistic mind as a weapon for super-detectives.

Despite the criticism of the trope, throughout the series, Abed does catch numerous details that his friends miss, leading to identification of impostors, manipulative plans, and other plots that might go overlooked. As is often the case with

Community, it's not always clear whether the show is celebrating or criticizing a trope, or possibly both simultaneously.

When the Swedish/Danish series *The Bridge (Bron/Broen)* was released in 2011, it became an international hit. One of the most successful versions of Scandinoir on television, the show's central character, Saga Norén (Sofia Helin), is widely seen as autistic, but as is often the case, this possibility is never discussed on the show. The series opens with a corpse found on the Øresund Bridge linking Denmark and Sweden, found exactly on the border between the two nations. The Swedish Saga, who demonstrates many classic autistic traits in her social interactions, is partnered with Martin Rohde from Denmark, an outgoing individual. Throughout their investigations, their differing personalities both complement and clash.

The series ran for four seasons, featuring a new case each season, with a growing focus on Saga's past and how it shaped her and threatened her future. The show has been adapted into an American version (2013-2014), set between the United States and Mexico, starring Diane Kruger as the American Detective Sonya Cross. The first of two seasons follows the original show closely, going off onto an original plotline for the second and final season. *The Tunnel* (2013-2017), transporting the action to the United Kingdom and France, starred Clémence Poésy as Elise Wassermann, a French policewoman. Like the American production, *The Tunnel* mirrors the first season of the original show before creating new storylines for the next two series. All three characters exhibit autistic tendencies, but notably, in the special features to the first season's DVD, the makers of *The Tunnel* state that they were trying to "move away" from autism in their depiction of Elise. As Saga, Sonya, and Elise all have strong similarities yet very different character arcs, they will be analyzed both in a group and separately. Though the series has been adapted for Austrian-German, Russian-Estonian, Malaysian-Singaporean, and Grecian-Turkish settings, as these versions are to the best of my knowledge not available for English-language viewers, and in at least one case, did not endow autistic characteristics upon the female lead, they will not be discussed here.

Since its publication in 2003, *The Curious Incident of the Dog in the Night-Time* by Mark Haddon has become a runaway bestseller, and it has done much to bring autism to the public eye, though with this success and acclaim has come a share of controversy as well. A film version of the novel has languished in development limbo for over a decade, but a stage adaptation by Simon Stephens has swept theater awards and become a major hit, and as the original production was filmed for National Theatre Live, it will be discussed here. In this 2012 production, Christopher is portrayed by Luke Treadaway.

Christopher John Francis Boone is the central character, a fifteen-year-old in England with a talent for mathematics. He presents with numerous autistic tendencies, though his condition is not specified in the book, and Haddon has on occasion avoided pinning a label of Christopher's condition, even when publishers, promotors, and critics have been more certain in diagnosing Christopher. As the book begins, Christopher is grieving the recent loss of his mother, and his quiet neighborhood is shocked by the brutal killing of his neighbor's dog. A suspect himself, Christopher decides to investigate the canine's slaying, and along the way, his focus shifts to finding out what really happened to his mother. Along the way, he's forced to push himself far beyond his comfort zone, trying to navigate a world that often strikes him as being hostile and confusing.

The 2013-2015 series *Hannibal* was a reimagining of Thomas Harris's Hannibal Lecter novels, save for *The Silence of the Lambs*, where, due to rights issues, none of the events or the characters first introduced in that novel could be mentioned. Hugh Dancy stars as Will Graham, the criminal profiler whose ability to place himself into the psyches of brutal killers often takes him to some very dark mental places. Graham only appeared in the first Lecter novel, *Red Dragon*. In this series, however, the first two seasons contain numerous original plotlines and characters, with the first season shaped around the hunt for the serial killer Garrett Jacob Hobbes, nicknamed "The Minnesota Shrike" (this is a fleeting reference from the novel *Red Dragon*). Numerous callouts to the other books fill the series, including *The Silence of the Lambs* references that are sufficiently vague or general so as not to violate copyright. The first half of the third and final season is a reworking of *Hannibal and Hannibal Rising*, and the second half is an expanded adaptation of *Red Dragon*.

As the television series opens, Graham works for the FBI as a consultant, visiting crime scenes in order to provide profiles of particularly brutal killers. Graham calls his profiling process "interpreting the evidence." Upon arriving at a crime scene, after a quick examination of the area, he is able to determine exactly how the violent act was committed, and replicate the mind of the person who committed the crime. In the premiere episode, "Apéritif" (S1E1), Graham discusses his analytic abilities with his supervisor at the FBI, Jack Crawford.

CRAWFORD. Where do you fall on the spectrum?
GRAHAM. My horse is hitched to a post that is closer to Asperger's and autistics than narcissists and sociopaths.

CRAWFORD. But you can empathize with narcissists and sociopaths.
GRAHAM. I can empathize with anybody. It's less to do with a personality disorder than an active imagination.

The controversy over the characterization of Graham as having a form of autism will be discussed later, in the chapter on autism. For now, it should be noted that Graham's profiling skills lead him to work with the then-respected psychiatrist Dr. Hannibal Lecter, and the central relationship of the show is between the two men, as they begin as friends solving crimes together, only for Graham's psyche to be seriously shaken in part due to exposure to the evil close to him, though it takes him a while to determine the source of the danger. Over the course of the three seasons, Graham has to deal with his own increasingly slippery grasp of morality and his uncomfortably tenuous hold on his own sanity.

The short-lived 2013 series *King & Maxwell*, based on the book series by David Baldacci, stars two neurotypical ex-Secret Service agents, Sean King (Jon Tenney) and Michelle Maxwell (Rebecca Romijn), now running a private investigative agency. In the first episode, they meet Edgar Roy (Ryan Hurst), an autistic man with brilliant analytical skills. Roy spent nearly a decade in a fact-checking government job before transferring to a secret position at a corporation specializing in military matters, until he was arrested on suspicion of being a serial killer. After Roy's defense lawyer (a buddy of King's) is murdered, King and Maxwell investigate and prove Roy's innocence, discovering that he was framed by a rival company to discredit his employer in the hopes of taking over government contracts. It is never made clear why Roy was not reinstated to his former job back after he was vindicated, or why his former employer was not sued and forced to compensate him for wrongful termination, or why comparable litigation was not launched against those who set him up for crimes he did not commit.

In need of a new job, Roy starts working for King and Maxwell, and despite some initial trepidation about hiring him, the pair finds Roy to be a valuable asset, and his technological and information-organizing skill soon prove vital to their investigations. For his part, Roy quickly bonds with his new employers and their associate, an ostensibly reformed counterfeiter named Benny (Dichen Lachman), and though his quirks, such as neatly arranging items and excess literalism, often nonplus his colleagues, they steadily grow to like and trust him.

On the four-episode 2014 British series *Chasing Shadows*, everybody who meets the central character, DS Sean Stone (Reece Shearsmith), realizes at once that he does not think or behave like most people. However, he has no official autism diagnosis, and his co-workers instead categorize him as being rude and difficult. His blunt honesty and self-recriminations at a press conference create a public relations embarrassment, and despite his skill as an investigator, he's demoted and sent to the Missing Persons department, which is meant to be career purgatory. There, he reluctantly partners with Ruth Hattersley (Alex Kingston), a civilian analyst who, in a typical case of crafting yin-yang characters, is skilled at connecting with other people. Over the course of a pair of two-part mysteries, they have a tense relationship due to Stone's inability to forge a connection, but they manage to catch a pair of multiple murderers – Stone despises the term "serial killer," because he thinks the term glamourizes the homicidal.

Despite some grudging respect for Stone's skills, his superior officer and other colleagues are constantly frustrated by him, and he's generally disliked. The only people who show Stone genuine affection are his part-time housekeeper, who does her best to encourage him to improve his social skills, and her young daughter. Stone seems truly unable to understand why his behavior might cause other people to be hostile towards him. He has a strong sense of justice, displays uncontrolled fury at lying, and he exhibits many classic autistic characteristics, such as retreating to a closet to sit and stim when he's upset.

The series ends on a cliffhanger, and it's possible that the show was cancelled before planned storylines could further explore Stone's psyche. Other than a passing reference from Hattersley about the possibility that Stone may have some sort of psychological condition, no one cares enough to explore why he acts as he does. Stone is simply the target of undisguised frustration and annoyance, with no one trying to understand him.

The Canadian series *Murdoch Mysteries* (2008-present) is a historical crime comedy series set in Toronto. The show begins in 1895 (perhaps a reference to the famous poem noting that at 221B Baker Street, it is "always 1895."), and advances one year each season. The title character, William Murdoch (Yannick Bisson), is a brilliant detective and scientist who creates inventions to help solve cases, often using anachronistic flashes of brilliance. Indeed, due to his occasional discomfort in social situations, obsessive focus with his scientific pursuits, and occasionally excessive formality, some fans have wondered if Murdoch himself shows mild autistic symptoms. Another detective who joined the series a decade into the show's run exhibits more obvious symptoms.

Llewellyn Watts (Daniel Maslany), first appears on the long-running series in Season 10's "Concocting a Killer," where he's called to investigate after a man Murdoch sent to prison years earlier is released in the light of new evidence. Watts is tasked with determining if and how Murdoch went wrong. Understandably, Murdoch is initially hostile to Watts, but as the investigation progresses, the two come to like and respect each other, and Watts becomes a recurring character, solving cases alongside Murdoch and the rest of his team.

Watts has no filter, often saying things that are not meant negatively, but could be misinterpreted by people depending on their moods. An intellectual, he often muses on philosophical matters, and he has a distinct gait and a love for the city's ethnic street foods. He was orphaned at a young age and looked after by his sister for a while before she vanished, leaving him to spend much of his life trying to find her. Though he displays attraction to women in some of his earlier appearances, by season thirteen his romantic interests are suddenly directed solely towards males. Due to the early loss of his family, he grew up unaware that he was Jewish.

Watts displays many classic autistic attributes, and his offbeat behavior and awkwardness often cause comment from his peers, but given the time period, it's not surprising that no one has a name for his brain function. Though the term "autism" wouldn't be used, it's certainly possible that *Murdoch Mysteries*, a series that delights in anticipating technology, trends, and ideas many decades before their actual emergence, might choose to create an early study of autism and give it a different name, much like "serial killers," a term not used until the 1970s, are referred to as "sequential killers" on the show. As the central character of Dr. Julia Ogden (Hélène Joy), Murdoch's eventual wife, is trained in psychiatry, it is certainly possible that in a future season, the show might explore autism long before the subject was widely studied (and better understood) in real life, though using different terminology.

Detective Sweet is a 2016 Chinese series, also released under the translated title *Miss Sugar Holmes*, though the parallels to Conan Doyle do not appear to be nearly as pronounced as in *Miss Sherlock* and *IQ 246*. As it has not yet received a dubbed or English-subtitled version to date, I cannot properly analyze the series, but it should be mentioned for the sake of completeness, and though the dialogue is inaccessible to me, I can describe what I have seen on YouTube. Su Teng (Chen Xiao Ping) is a young woman with autism, who is first shown waiting for public transportation, looking around her and playing with a 4x4 Rubik's Cube. Soon after she solves the puzzle, the vehicle runs over the side of a cliff, but she survives. Somehow, the crash altered her brain, making her super-smart and incredibly observant. It goes without saying that I certainly do not recommend that people with autism get into car accidents in the hopes of accentuating their observational powers. Disregarding the realism of the story, Su Teng begins working with the police to solve crimes.

Created by Stephen King, Holly Gibney entered the world as a supporting character in a trilogy of novels. She met the retired police officer Bill Hodges in *Mr. Mercedes* while he was trying to solve a case he hadn't been able to crack – a mass murderer who had plowed a Mercedes into a crowd of people. Midway through the investigation, Bill starts dating one of Holly's relatives, and after a tragedy, Holly joins Bill's investigation and the two become partners in private detection. In the books, Bill Hodges passes away at the close of the trilogy, *End of Watch*, and Holly continues solving cases on her own. Notably, while the first season is quite realistic, later seasons include more supernatural aspects, and in Holly's post-Bill investigative career, she tends to deal with inexplicable, malignant preternatural forces. The three-season series *Mr. Mercedes*, follows the first book reasonably faithfully in the first season, and heavily alters and rearranges the events of the next two books for seasons two and three.

On the 2017-2019 show *Mr. Mercedes,* Holly (Justine Lupe) appears midway through the season. In her first appearance, she's clearly distraught, and has been given unspecified treatment in the past for her mental state, but her therapy hasn't helped her too much – she's highly uncomfortable in social situations, and her stern mother treats her as a naughty child when Holly gets upset. Holly is very smart, sweet, and kind, but she responds badly to numerous stimuli, demonstrating many of the classic autistic behaviors and reactions. As she gets to know Bill and starts doing detective work, she gradually builds confidence and becomes better at dealing with other people. An inheritance sets her on the way to full independence, and by the series' end, she's a very capable private investigator, routinely stands up for herself, and takes pleasure in helping others. While her condition *improves*, it never *vanishes*, and while she's made giant strides in functionality, she can still be left stimming uncontrollably at the prospect of a stressful situation. In *Mr. Mercedes*, Holly illustrates how a supportive network of people and the opportunity to use one's strengths in a useful manner can have a positive effect on a person with autism.

Cynthia Erivo took on the role in the 2020 series *The Outsider*, which was made by a separate production team from *Mr. Mercedes*. The showrunner changed *The Outsider's* version of Holly in several distinct ways in order to distinguish her from the other series, and even considered changing the character's name, but King rejected this proposal. Erivo's take on Holly is slightly more muted than Lupe's, though her idiosyncrasies, insights, and competence are essentially the same. Aside from appearance and wardrobe, the main difference between the two is that Erivo's Holly is fully independent from the beginning and though occasionally upset, appears calmer and almost never seems likely to have a debilitating meltdown. In contrast, Lupe's Holly was often doing well but often gave signs that she had to struggle and strive to maintain her equilibrium. While Lupe's Holly is accepted and loved by her colleagues, the cast of *The Outsider* is constantly befuddled by Erivo's Holly, as the other characters have trouble seeing past her downplayed idiosyncrasies. Indeed, the title *The Outsider* refers not only to the murderous supernatural force, but also to Holly herself.

In the books and *Mr. Mercedes*, Holly has been prescribed Lexapro and takes it irregularly, and occasionally self-medicates with cigarettes. Additionally, Holly begins *The Outsider* on her own, lacking the circle of friends that proved so helpful to her wellbeing in *Mr. Mercedes*, though as she tries to track down a monstrous shape-shifting destructive force, the new collection of fellow investigators quickly bonds with her and comes to respect her. Lupe's Holly is a woman who is learning how to overcome a disability and use her mental wiring to her advantage. Erivo's Holly has distinct autistic tendencies, but she rarely seems hampered by them.

Astrid et Raphaëlle (2019-Present) is a French-Belgian series, sometimes called simply *Astrid* in English-speaking markets, but it also is renamed *Bright Minds* occasionally. Astrid Nielsen (Sara Mortensen) is a police archivist with autism. Raphaëlle Coste (Lola Dewaere), is a neurotypical police officer. Astrid has an extensive memory of the crimes in her files, and her knowledge consistently helps Raphaëlle close cases. Meanwhile, Raphaëlle provides Astrid with friendship and guidance in navigating the world. Unlike all of the other series in this study save *Detective Sweet*, I have not been able to view the entire show in translation, so only a small portion of the series factors into this analysis, and like *Detective Sweet*, the series is mentioned for the sake of completeness.

The 2020 movie *The Night Clerk* features an autistic character who barely qualifies as a detective, but rather maneuvers through a murder case rather than actually solves it. Still, given his actions and the role that his condition plays in his decisions, he is included in this analysis. In the film, Bart Bromley (Tye Sheridan) is a man with Asperger's Syndrome in his early twenties. He is smart, but his educational background is left unclear. He lives with his mother (Helen Hunt), who loves him deeply and accepts all of his idiosyncrasies and preferences, allowing him to spend most of his time in the basement, leaving his meals on the steps without face-to-face contact with him. Bart apparently got his job at a hotel's front desk due to a policy of hiring disabled people, but unsettlingly, he has set up video cameras in several of the rooms. Apparently this was not for prurient purposes, but instead was so he could observe other people and mimic their speech patterns and movements. Bart seems to have no idea that people might be less than enthusiastic about his invasion of their privacy.

One night, a woman checks into the hotel, and while Bart watches her from home through the camera, a figure whose face is conveniently just out of the camera's sight enters the room and fights with her. Bart rushes back to work and arrives just as the woman's shot to death. Possibly due to a misinterpretation of his mental state and some obvious inconstancies in his story, due to clumsy lies meant to cover up his hidden cameras, Bart becomes the chief suspect, and he's reluctant to release the video that can clear him – of murder, at least. When he's transferred to a different branch of the hotel chain and meets the beautiful Andrea (Ana de Armas), she's kind and understanding toward him, recognizing his condition, and Bart's immediately smitten. As the narrative progresses, Bart pursues Andrea, battles the police investigation, and tries to identify the real killer while figuring out what to do with his videos.

Throughout the movie, Bart's social awkwardness is always given center stage, and he seems to have no interest in modifying his reactions or questioning the morality of his actions in spying. His main thoughts of change are purely *external*, meant to make himself more attractive to Andrea. Viewers see little evidence of his wrestling with the moral issues of peeping or withholding information, and it's unclear why he turned to secret video cameras to learn other behaviors instead of seeking professional guidance. The identity of the killer is discovered through chance rather than investigation, and ultimately, Bart's psyche and deeper emotions are largely left unexplored.

Professor T is another series that has found new life in many countries. It began as a Belgian show (three seasons, 2015-2018), with Koen De Bouw as Professor Jasper Teerlinck, and adapted versions set in Germany, France, and the Czech Republic followed. Due to language and availability issues, the British version (2021-Present), with Ben Miller as Professor Jasper Tempest, will be studied here. Professor Tempest is a highly skilled scholar of criminology at the University of Cambridge, and he is occasionally called upon to help the official police solve crimes. Despite his high intelligence, he has difficulty functioning due to his obsessive-compulsive disorder. As discussed previously with Adrian Monk and Dexter Morgan, being diagnosed with one condition does not necessarily preclude having another condition, and in an interview titled

"""*Professor T*" Star Ben Miller: "I Was Born to Play This Part,""" Miller has explained that he views his character as being autistic as well.

The last character to be profiled here is also one of the few to receive an official diagnosis in the context of the television show. *Extraordinary Attorney Woo* is a 2022 South Korean series starring Park Eun-bin as Woo Young-woo, a recent law school graduate with autism. Largely nonverbal for most of her early years, Woo Young-woo demonstrated the ability to read, understand, and memorize complex legal principles from a very young age. As an adult, she reached the top of her law school class, but was unable to find a job due to her disability. It's not until the CEO of the law firm Hanbada secretly intervenes that she's given a chance to show off her legal skills.

Woo Young-woo insists on wearing soft fabrics that stand apart from her colleagues' more traditional business attire, wears headphones in public to drown out distracting ambient noise, compulsively introduces herself with the same opening spiel, eats her favorite food kimbap (rice and various fillings, rolled up in a seaweed wrapper and sliced) whenever possible, and has intense reactions to various stimuli and situations, often needing a few seconds to mentally prepare before she enters a room or uses a revolving door. Additionally, she is fascinated by whales, filling her room with whale imagery, sharing her encyclopedic autodidactic knowledge of whales with people even when they have zero interest in the subject, and when she has an epiphany about a case, she pictures a whale in her mind. One season has aired as of this writing, but a second is in production. Over the course of the first sixteen episodes, Woo Young-woo improves her courtroom skills, builds relationships and friendships with her colleagues, dates for the first time, and finds new ways to deal with stressors and use her brain functions to the advantage of both herself and her clients.

Given the popularity and the critical response to the show, as of this writing, several countries including the United States have remakes of *Extraordinary Attorney Woo* in development. Concerns over maintaining the charm and quality of the original series notwithstanding, it will be interesting to see how other countries address the presentation of autism.

Once again, the purpose of these essays is not to prove that the characters discussed here officially have autism. The goal of these essays *is to use the characterizations in the analyzed productions in order to provide a resource for people with autism to explain their condition to others.* Explaining the autistic experience to others is a challenging undertaking, and though no single performance will be a useful parallel for everybody, this combined analysis will hopefully be useful in starting a conversation on portrayals of autism. In addition, stereotypes, tropes, oversimplifications, and controversies regarding these portrayals will be analyzed, as I look at some of the shortcomings that arise from these dramatizations, and how future productions might rectify or at least address these issues.

This list is not necessarily completev– there are bound to be other examples that I have missed, and some possibilities which are more controversial. In some cases, there are only vague hints that a detective may be on the spectrum, such as in *Queens of Mystery*, (2019– Present), where Jane Stone (Siobhan Redmond), one of a trio of mystery-writing, crime-solving sisters, features some of the quirks and abilities often associated with autism, such as the ability to detect sounds no one hears and a remarkable memory for numbers, but these characteristics are so minimally developed that I did not feel comfortable placing her on this list officially.*

Ultimately, quality literature and drama create a bond between the work and the person appreciating it. By engaging with unfamiliar characters, situations, and ideas, readers or viewers can enhance their understanding of what might otherwise be completely foreign to them. I also hope to share my own experiences, illustrating how certain productions and actor portrayals have been invaluable in helping me explain my own autistic reactions and struggles to others. Because this topic is so personal to me, I had great difficulty in writing it. Normally, I am able to produce analytical critiques fairly swiftly, but because every character and incident discussed here causes me to flash back to times that were particularly challenging for me, writing came exponentially more slowly. I hope that the results are useful to people, both for those with autism, and for those who know and care about them, and that these essays help to facilitate explanations and understanding.

---

* After the completion of this manuscript, the television series *Elsbeth* (2024), starring Carrie Preston as an attorney widely seen as being on the autism spectrum, premiered. The character of Elsbeth Tascioni originated on *The Good Wife* and also appeared on its spin-off *The Good Fight*. In *Elsbeth*, the title character moves to New York City and solves mysteries there. Since as of this writing, only one episode of *Elsbeth* has aired, it will not be included in this analysis, though if there is a revised and updated edition of this book in the future, *Elsbeth* will almost certainly be included in it.

CHAPTER THREE
Autism: The Condition That Must Not Be Named

Hardly any of the sleuths discussed here have official diagnoses of autism. Astrid in *Astrid et Raphaëlle* and the titular *Extraordinary Attorney Woo* have received diagnoses from independent mental health professionals. But in almost every other case, the word "autism" is either never mentioned or the possibility of the sleuth being autistic is only mentioned once or twice, and never explored in-depth. Why are screenwriters so reluctant to come right out and state that a character has autism?

Lacking the opportunity to interview these screenwriters, the best that can be done is to analyze the information that is provided on-screen. In some cases, it makes perfect sense that words like "autism" and "Asperger's" are absent from the characters' vocabulary. In the period pieces, such as the Downey *Sherlock Holmes* and *Murdoch Mysteries*, it is quite logical that no one would use that terminology. In fact, it would be anachronistic if such words were used, for although the term "autism" was coined in the late nineteenth century, it would not have been applied at that time to characters like Sherlock Holmes, Llwellyn Watts, and William Murdoch.

In *The Curious Incident of the Dog in the Night-Time*, Christopher Boone is identified as having a mental disability, but it's never expressly stated in the script that he has a form of autism. The debate over Christopher's precise mental state and the authors' presentation of it has been hotly debated, and this study will not go into that controversy, but it will take note of this deliberate ambiguity.

At times, a character may be *suspected* to have autism, but such references are fleeting, and they almost never come as a result of a qualified professional. Will Graham in *Hannibal* diagnoses himself, the titular *Doc Martin* has a doctor suggest the possibility of being on the spectrum but the issue is never addressed again, Cumberbatch's Sherlock has Doctor Watson suggest Asperger's but never makes sure his friend has a proper diagnosis, and others, like Abed Nadir on *Community* or Spencer Reid on *Criminal Minds*, simply listen to a non-professional pronounce a diagnosis and never seek official confirmation.

Mostly, the characters discussed in this study simply behave in a manner that they find natural, and those around them tend to respond with puzzlement, offense, and mockery. Most of these characters suspected of having autism are aware to varying extents that they think and feel differently from the vast majority of the population, but without knowing that there is a condition that affects them, they either remain unchanged, or are compelled to devise their own ways of overcoming any difficulties they may have.

There are certain thematic consequences of avoiding official autism diagnoses. By not providing the characters with an official diagnosis, many of the characters are denied the opportunity to seek help for any difficulties they may experience. Saga on *The Bridge*, for example, is fully aware that she isn't "normal," to use her own words in Season Two. She knows that she has difficulties with relationships and connecting with people, but she never expresses frustration or sorrow over it. She does, however, strive to improve her interactive skills, starting in the second season, based on a study plan she designed for herself of reading books and speaking to others, though she soon believes that her program isn't doing her much good.

It should be noted that a few of these characters do not appear to be suffering unduly from their autism. Temperance Brennan on *Bones*, for example, has an exceptionally strong personal and professional life. Most of the other detectives have at least a successful career, and a few others have strong work-life balances. Many of these characters never have meltdowns, never fear for their own sanity, and never display any angst over any perceived differences between themselves and other people.

Also notable is the fact that many of the characters *do* receive treatment by mental health professionals, but at no point do any of these therapists suggest autism as a possible diagnosis. Were these shows created twenty or thirty years ago, the absence of such terminology would be understandable, but at this point in time, it seems as though the absolute refusal to categorically declare that a character has autism is deliberate, and that the showrunners wish to avoid wandering into such express categorization.

Cumberbatch's Sherlock briefly sees a mental health professional in the fourth series after a case goes tragically wrong, but this very short scene is devoted to his grief and guilt rather than labelling his mental processes, though a modern psychologist ought to have recognized the symptoms.

Some characters are forced into counseling for the sake of their jobs. In the fourth and final season of *The Bridge (Bron/Broen)*, Saga Norén is compelled to see a doctor after being released from prison after being wrongly convicted of murder. The therapy is supposed to help her return to work, though her doctor trains her to me more flexible in her worldview and to leave her job as a police officer in search of a fresher, more fulfilling career. Comparably, Robert Goren reluctantly sees a therapist in the tenth and final season of *Law & Order: Criminal Intent* as a condition of his reinstatement. Temperance Brennan is sporadically compelled by the FBI to see a psychiatrist in order to improve her then-working relationship with her partner Seeley Booth and works closely with the FBI psychologist Lance Sweets (John Francis Daley). Will Graham on *Hannibal* is required to see the titular Dr. Lecter after shooting a suspect, but Lecter's machinations are designed to twist Graham's psyche rather than repair it.

Others seek help voluntarily. Adrian Monk regularly attends therapy in order to combat his numerous phobias. The titular Doctor Martin's lack of an official diagnosis particularly strains credulity, as in the later series, he not only sees a couples therapist who stays current with the medical literature, but he is also close to his Aunt Ruth (Eileen Atkins), an expert in psychology. Furthermore, his own wife Louisa trains as a child therapist by the series' end, and one could safely assume that she'd be taught to look out for autism. Professor T. enters therapy in the second series in order to deal with his social issues and anxiety. In *Murdoch Mysteries*, Murdoch's eventual wife Julia trains as a psychiatrist, and he occasionally discusses issues with her, and on one occasion Watts consults with Julia as well for his personal troubles.

Still others of the characters discussed here enter therapy through circumstance. Dexter Morgan initially sees a sinister psychiatrist in the first season's "Shrink Wrap" (S1E8), not initially as a desire for self-improvement, but to vet the doctor because he correctly suspects him of deliberately driving patients to suicide. In the eighth season, Dr. Evelyn Vogel, the woman who set him up to be a serial killer by glorifying psychopaths and encouraged the murder of killers as a means of treatment, re-enters his life and provides dubious guidance as to how he should deal with his blood lust and relationships. For Lisbeth Salander, therapy was a traumatic experience, as the uncaring court system forced her into a mental hospital where she was abused by her doctor.

This list illustrates how all of these characters had access to mental health professionals, but the topic of autism never arises. Of course, the therapists are all fictional characters and cannot be blamed for their failure to diagnose another fictional character. It's the writers who made a conscious choice to provide their detectives with autistic attributes, but not for them to be openly addressed. While their reasons for doing so must remain theoretical based on the available information, it's notable that so many shows create autistic-presenting characters but steadfastly refuse to diagnose them.

To give an example of how a lack of a proper diagnosis can affect even a seemingly successful autistic person negatively, an instance from *Bones* will be critiqued. At the start of *Bones'* run, the show broke the usual template by crafting an episode that was focused more on the title character and how others viewed her than it was about the solution to the crime. Rather than spending the whole episode trying to track down a murderer's identity, the guilty party is caught early on, and the lion's share of the episode is devoted to the trial of the culprits, and the very real possibility that they might be acquitted due to how the jurors respond to Bones' personality.

As the episode opens, Bones' former professor– and lover– Michael Stires (Josh Hopkins) comes to town for a job interview, leading to a resumption of their relationship. Booth drops off a new corpse to be examined, a young woman who was concealed inside a refrigerator. After an examination, a brief investigation reveals that the victim was a supposed kidnapping victim who was never found after ransom negotiations went nowhere. Surprisingly quickly, Bones and Booth learn that the victim was an opioid addict and that her doctor's former office manager helped provide her with pills. The detectives soon find proof that the ex-office manager and her boyfriend were responsible, holding her hostage and doping her into compliance until they accidentally gave her a lethal dose.

But the show does not end there. As the trial begins, Stires takes a job as a defense witness and starts challenging all of Bones' conclusions. When it's time for Bones to take the stand, she uses a great deal of technical language and presents the details dispassionately, causing the jurors to not only be bored by her testimony, but also to judge her as being cold and clinical. Stires, in contrast, oozes charm and quickly wins over the jurors, arguing that instead of a malicious kidnapping, the victim's wounds and death were due to sex games gone wrong and an accidental recreational drug overdose. He also delivers numerous not-so-subtle digs at Bones, sniping that she's wedded to her preconceived notions, and that her arrogance blinds her to other interpretations of the evidence. Bones is livid, as Stires is ignoring the evidence in an unprofessional manner, using contemptuous aspersions and force of personality instead of solid scientific analysis, but the jury is firmly on Stires' side.

In order to win them over, Booth convinces the prosecutor to ask Bones questions about why she became a forensic anthropologist, and segues into the disappearance of her parents and how that affected her. As Bones responds to the questions, she's visibly rattled, and for the first time, the jurors see her display emotions and learn more about her as a person. By the time her second round of testimony is finished, the jurors have grown sympathetic towards Bones, and the defendants are convicted. Disgusted with Stires, Bones breaks up with him, and she's initially livid with Booth for telling the prosecutor about those aspects of her past. A minute later, though, at the episode's end, she concedes the effectiveness of Booth's strategy in getting justice, and she forgives Booth.

The title of the episode, "The Girl in the Fridge," has a double meaning. Ostensibly, it refers to the crime victim, the young woman who was tied up, fed painkillers until she overdosed, and then her corpse was shoved into a refrigerator and dumped like garbage. But there's a second meaning, one where "The Girl" refers to Bones, and "the Fridge" is a metaphor for the way people who do not know her well view her. This "Fridge" is her just-the-facts attitude, which people interpret as cold and unfeeling. This is a classic case of people expecting everybody else to act and emote in exactly the same way that they would. Bones believes that the facts should speak for themselves, but makes no effort to use layman's terms. She therefore is considered as being arrogant, talking down to the jurors. While Bones treats the victim as a subject of study, when Booth, Hodgins, and Angela take the stand, they all present themselves as professionals with hearts, all humanizing and sympathizing with the victim. None of them are adopting a false persona, and Bones sees no reason why she should pretend to be anybody but her natural personality, either.

In fairness, Bones is guilty of the same attitude as the jurors: expecting others to behave and react exactly like she does. Just as the jurors judge her for not displaying emotion in the way that they think is proper, Bones condemns them for not being sufficiently focused on the facts, weighing the evidence empirically and dispassionately. The jury does not understand Bones, and she fails to understand them. Bones expects the jury to conform to her expectations and vice-versa. She cannot accept that most people's thought processes differ from her own.

Throughout the episode, those who know Bones best know at once that her distinctive personality is in no way a detriment to her job or their affection for her. Upon watching the comparably neuroatypical-presenting laboratory assistant Zack Addy trying and failing to fist-bump Bones, Angela says "I love it when you two impersonate earthlings." There's no malice in Angela's statement, and there are no external expressions of offense from Bones and Zack. Later, after Bones is smarting after being rebuked for her testimony Bones' supervisor, Dr. Daniel Goodman, tells her that "You have many skills, Temperance, not one of them includes communicating with the average person on the street... which is exactly what juries are made of." He informs her that Stires also applied for the job Bones eventually received at the Smithsonian, but despite Stires' lengthier résumé, Goodman correctly concluded that Bones was the superior scientist.

This adds another twist to Stires' actions. Though he did not realize he would have the opportunity when he first visited Bones, he had no compunction about going on the witness stand and insulting and humiliating his paramour. His denigration of her was in part a reaction to the narcissistic injury of her beating him out for a job. Later on, he acts as if a smile from him is enough to convince Bones to forget all of the sneers in his testimony, and that they will resume their relationship as if nothing had happened.

This characterization is a demonstration that people with autism are not the only ones who can be totally blind to other people's thoughts and feelings. Bones and Stires make for an interesting comparative duality. The jurors see Bones as cold and rather inhuman in her clinical approach to testifying. In reality, Bones is no emotionless android. She cares deeply for her friends, she is passionate about her work, and she has a very strong ethical code. It is not that she does not have emotions, she just shows them in a different way from how the average person would expect.

The same cannot be said for Stires, who presents himself as an amiable charmer, and initially comes across as so likable that he wins over the jurors without offering justification for his supposed scientific conclusions. Perhaps his career successes were due more to similarly superficial charm, and he was passed over when perceptive people like Goodman saw through his veneer. Stires' actions show he has no respect for Bones as a person or a forensic anthropologist, but he still wants to have sex with her, as if she is so susceptible to his advances that every insult would be instantly forgotten. Just as it's hazardous to identify fictional characters as autistic, it's similarly troublesome to try to pin an official personality disorder on Stires, but even the American Psychological Association would probably accept the statement that he's a jerk. When people first meet Stires, they are initially won over by his good looks and charm. As his actions in this episode prove, he's a whitewashed sepulcher. The apple with the shiniest peel is rotten underneath.

"The Girl in the Fridge" is a cautionary tale. Presentations of emotion often connected to autism may create false impressions, and unpleasant people may be skilled at faking amiability. But while the mask can slip off people like Stires through their selfish actions, it is harder to learn what people with autism are truly like until one actually gets to know them. And if the autistic person is reluctant to open up about very private matters, or if someone isn't there to help explain the autistic person's true character, then there's nothing to correct the misconceptions. Of course, this doesn't just apply to the autistic. The moral of "The Girl in the Fridge" is that one cannot judge anybody on first impressions alone. Until one knows more about that person and that individual's formative influences, holding that person to one's own standards of behavior is bound to create a distorted picture of that person's true nature.

Moving on to other professional women with autism, the two characters with an official diagnosis, Astrid Nielsen and Woo Young-woo, have the benefit of knowing why their minds react as they do, and they can take steps to help themselves function better. Astrid attends group therapy, asks Raphaëlle for advice, and devises plans to help with dating and other interactions. Woo Young-woo, by contrast, does not receive professional help or guidance, (the implication being that financial concerns prevent fuller treatment) and instead depends mostly upon her own preferred tactics, such as noise-cancelling headphones and counting to three before entering a room, in order to function in the outside world.

  The effects of not having terminology to describe a condition are explored in *The Outsider* when Cythia Erivo's Holly Gibney is introduced in S1E3 – "Dark Uncle." When an investigative team hires Holly to probe a seemingly impossible alibi, the individuals who are previously acquainted with Holly warn Ralph Anderson (Ben Mendelsohn), that she is "unique." After explaining some of her amazing mental abilities and demonstrating some personal idiosyncrasies, Erivo's Holly explains how when she was a child and exhibited very distinctive behavior, her parents took her to countless specialists, who performed batteries of tests. Despite being analyzed by the best members of their fields, they had no explanation to define the workings of her brain. Her condition, then, is "inexplicable."

  A lawyer, Harold Salomon (Bill Camp) speaks highly of Holly's investigative skills, but immediately calls her mental stability into question. Having no name or explanation for her abilities or unconventional social comportment, Salomon turns to pejoratives. Sadly, it's not her memory or analytical skills that define Holly in Salomon's eyes, it's her quirks that smear her as a crazy person. And Salomon is not a fool or a cruel person. He's an intelligent attorney determined to prove his late client's innocence, and due to his dedication to his friend's memory, he's a strong and sympathetic character. Yet even this otherwise smart and likable person is so befuddled by Holly's inexplicable abilities that rather than focusing on her superpowers, he focuses not on her actual strengths, but on her perceived differences, which make her a befuddling oddity in most people's eyes rather than an awe-inspiring figure.

Certainly not all people with autism have abilities similar to Holly's, and it is definitely possible that there are other factors that affect her brainpower. The point is not that the showrunners and creative team erred by not explicitly calling Holly an autistic savant. The issue being focused upon here is the fact that a brilliant person can be belittled and marginalized because supposedly "normal" individuals don't have a word or even a concept for her other than "crazy." Atypical behavior becomes her defining attribute, and that is grossly unfair to Holly.

There is something unsettling about the reluctance of so many shows to address the issue of autism. By not categorizing these characters as having a recognized and diagnosable condition, they are instead slapped with far less sensitive labels by their perplexed peers, who dub them anything from "quirky" to "weird" to "cold." It is like the writers wanted to give these characters certain distinctive attributes and social challenges, but they are reluctant to provide them with a road map for assistance or improved understanding by their associates. The writers give them difficulties, and then make precious little effort, if any to suggest a viable means of assistance. Perhaps an unintended side effect of the tendency to avoid autism is the possibility that undiagnosed autistic viewers can watch these series, see aspects of themselves on-screen, and then not realize that they may be on the spectrum themselves, or believe that there is nothing to be done to help them or alleviate any problems they may have, and the best they can do is to learn to live with their condition.

CHAPTER FOUR
How Realistic is "Realism?"

This chapter's titular question has been raised in countless reviews, articles, and YouTube comments. In coverage of *The Curious Incident of the Dog in the Night-Time*, *Extraordinary Attorney Woo*, or any of the other shows discussed here, someone says that these portrayals of autism are "not realistic." Elsewhere, many of the characters discussed in this study have been similarly criticized, with some autistic people stating that portrayals like those described in this book are radically dissimilar to their own experiences.

One central problem with this attitude is that it fails to consider how different autistic minds can be. When people with autism state that one portrayal in the media is "not realistic," they often qualify that with the declaration than it does not match their personal experiences. In *The Autistic Brain*, Temple Grandin explains that for a long time, she believed that because she thinks primarily in the form of pictures, she believed that *all* autistic people minds must work similarly. It was not until she saw the reviews of her book on Amazon that she discovered comments from other people with autism, explaining that their mental imaging processes were quite different.

Ultimately, when some people claim that a certain fictional character's depiction of what it is like to have autism is not "realistic," what this generally means is that the portrayal does not match their personal experiences or those of an autistic person they know. And this is valid. The wide-ranging nature of the autistic experience means that no single person can possibly represent the entire group. There are endless examples in the media where characters of certain ethnic groups are widely criticized for perpetuating unfair stereotypes, while simultaneously, people of the group being portrayed declare that watching the show reminds them of their own families. There is no way to please everybody all of the time, and a characterization that some people find hackneyed or offensive may be representative and relatable to others.

People with autism have just as wide-ranging levels of intelligence as neurotypical people, and certainly not everybody on the spectrum is cut out to be a detective. I deeply sympathize with autistic people who, in addition to the problems and limitations brought about by their brain wiring, have to deal with the inquiries of individuals with an incomplete understanding of how autism works, and ask questions like "Why aren't you a genius?" It adds insult to injury, as people who already wrestle with difficulties handling certain common tasks and situations have their troubles compounded by misguided expectations. Certainly the claim bandied about in certain circles that "autism is a superpower" is a radical oversimplification of how this form of brain function works. For many people, watching autistic savant characters can be hurtful because it feels like they received all of the negative aspects of autism without any of the supposed benefits. Social awkwardness, constant overstimulation, and reliance on rigid routines are hard enough to cope with on a daily basis when other people have an unjustified expectation, based upon popular culture, that all autistic people have incredible mental abilities.

A primary reason for writing this book is that in my personal case, many of the depictions discussed here *are an extremely accurate though incomplete depiction of my personal experiences with autism.* As will be explained later, many of these depictions mirror my own mental processes with uncanny accuracy. But many, perhaps most, possibly even the vast majority of people with autism have intensely different reactions from my own. So why, then, has the popular conception of the autistic mind so often been portrayed on-screen as exceptionally intelligent, preternaturally observant, and possessing incredible powers of memory? Certainly the entertainment industry has always been attracted to the most dramatic possible characterizations. The idea of people wired to have preternatural mental powers is irresistible to many screenwriters, and as is often the case, nuance is often lost and misconceptions can proliferate in the creation of fictional characters. But the fact that the "autistic super sleuth" trope has surged in popularity must be taken in tandem with the fact that people with brain patterns and thoughts exhibited by the characters discussed here do indeed exist, and there is nothing wrong with having stories about people like them told.

    I believe that the backlash to the savant portrayals of autistic people is unfair. While different forms of autism should certainly be portrayed in the media, the calls to abolish "autistic savant" characters are in themselves an attempt to limit the complexity of the public understanding of how autism works. Certainly more characters with autism who exhibit different mindsets, reactions, and behaviors would be a welcome development. However, some issues connected to these current limitations are connected to the fact that the general public and the entertainment industry are just a little bit behind the mental health profession in their knowledge of autism. It is only in the last few decades that research into autism has started to explore the breadth and depth of what it means to be autistic. Not too long ago, the idea of an "autistic spectrum" amongst mental health professionals would have met with incredulity, even scorn in some circles.

    Previously, I mentioned the Father Brown method and how it helped me with my interactions with other people. I believe that studying and critiquing dramatic portrayals of autism is a useful tool in helping people with autism explain their condition. Even when they personally are quite different from the depiction, the dramatization can be helpful in starting a conversation. People with autism can explain what comes closest to their own experiences, and what is far off the mark.

The goal of this book is to open up a means of communication and explanation. For people like me, shows like *Sherlock* and *Extraordinary Attorney Woo* and the stage production of *The Curious Incident of the Dog in the Night-Time* have proven to be invaluable tools for demonstrating to family members and friends how I think and react to the world. And I also believe that these portrayals can be just as useful to people with autism when they use them to explain how their own mental processes *differ* from what's on-screen.

One reason why I am fascinated by the fictional detectives discussed in this study is that I can see myself reflected in them. Part of my desire to write this book is also a need to *defend* them. In particular, I wish to respond to other critics who label them as unrealistic and ultimately harmful stereotypes, or, in the parlance of a frequently used remark, "a dumb screenwriter's conception of what a smart person is like." In real life and on-screen, when a person with autism deviates outside the accepted norms for behavior, they are often belittled and chastised like naughty children. They may be lambasted for causing offense, when they had no idea that their comments could be viewed as insulting. They may be denounced for being insensitive by people who assume that a certain understanding of societal expectations is universally inherent, thus, the atypical are forced to figure out how to behave through painful trial and error. In many cases, the characters shown here are viewed as insensitive jerks, unsettling oddballs, and weird annoyances, all because they do not fit a standard that does not suit their natural personality. In short, people with autism may be penalized for violating societal rules while the referees refuse to provide them with a copy of the rule book.

This book is not just for people with autism. It is also for those people who may not understand how their expectations of the autistic may be unrealistic, patronizing, and even cruel. In many cases, the neurotypical can be even more insensitive and insulting to the autistic than the autistic are to those they inadvertently offend or estrange. One of the goals of this book is to point out how many negative stereotypes about people with autism apply equally well to neurotypicals. When many people envision autism, all they see is a collection of idiosyncrasies and difficulties interacting socially. *Externals* understandably are more obvious to others than *internals*. But many of these supposed qualities are present in all kinds of people, and many people with autism do not present with stereotypical behaviors. Much of autism is a matter of mental processes, reactions and emotions – constructs that require creativity and artistic license to present effectively on-screen. The mental processes of the detectives studied in the book are not representative of all autistic people. But they are still worthy of study and helpful as a starting point for exploring and explaining the broader autistic spectrum.

CHAPTER FIVE
Autism: Born or Made?

Sometimes a blunt judgement is the only honest one. For decades, the prevailing wisdom on the nature and causes of autism in the mental health community was complete excrement.

Thorough histories of the study of autism have already been written, so only a brief summary of other works is necessary here. The term "autism" was first used in the early twentieth century, though certain mental processes connected to autism were studied decades before that, and it was in the middle of the century that the condition began to be explored more thoroughly, and it is only since the late decades of the twentieth century that the idea of a spectrum has been explored.

During the third quarter of the twentieth century, the self-proclaimed world expert on autism was Bruno Bettelheim, who promoted as fact the misguided theory that autism was not an inherent condition, but was damage inflicted by emotionally indifferent parenting, particularly cold and unfeeling mothers, who were slurred as "refrigerator mothers." This was based on perfunctory observations, over-generalizing, and possibly projection. Additionally, some of the parents might have had autism to varying degrees, thereby affecting their abilities to connect to their children. Bettelheim's influence and a credulous medical establishment lapped up the idea. The message was clear: If a child has autism, it's the mother's fault.

Much later, a study in the late twentieth century proclaimed a link between autism and vaccines, and this became accepted truth in many circles before later studies found no link and called the methodology of the early research into question. On the police drama *The Shield*, there was a very small subplot where the main character, Vic Mackey (Michael Chiklis) and his wife Corinne (Cathy Cahlin Ryan) discover that two of their young children have autism, and they angrily blame their doctor for harming their children through dangerous vaccines, equating a rise in autism with such medications. The counter-suggestion that autism has always existed medical professionals have simply learned how to spot it cuts little ice with the Mackeys, and autism is mentioned far less during the later seasons, but the subplot reflects the widespread misconceptions of the time.

Yet despite the debunking of the "refrigerator mother" and the vaccine theories, and the increased awareness of the potential genetic link to autism and other physiological factors causing it, nearly all of the autistic sleuths discussed in this study are portrayed as having traumas in their childhoods, including absent and/or emotionally aloof or abusive parents. Most screenwriters do not have training in autistic theory, and it seems that instead of simply attributing the characters' social awkwardness and other mental health issues to the autistic experience, they have to add a Freudian explanation as well, and it is implied that broken families and cold or overbearing mothers are to blame, at least in part, for the conditions of their children.

No information (or at least, hardly any) is given regarding the childhoods or parents of Downey's version of Sherlock Holmes, Chloe O'Brian, Grace Matsuki, Will Graham (aside from a fleeting mention that he never got a chance to know his mother), Edgar Roy, or Sean Stone on their respective television shows, but in almost every other case– save one– the characters come from broken families, and in many cases have neglectful, cold, or abusive parents, implying that at least in part, their condition is due to nurture, not nature.[1]

---

[1] Based on a lack of access to reliably translated versions of *Detective Sweet* and *Astrid*, they will be omitted from this chapter. Astrid's parents are characters in the series, but I have not been able to view any of the episodes

In virtually every instance, the sleuth in question is given a tragic backstory or difficult family relationship which can be extrapolated into the root cause for their social awkwardness or other behaviors that can present as symptoms of autism. These storylines ignore the likelihood that autism may have developed naturally in their brains, possibly due to genetics, and was not the result of trauma or abuse.

Remarkably, of the two dozen characters studied here, only one comes from an intact family with loving parents. That detective is Benedict Cumberbatch's Sherlock Holmes from *Sherlock*. In the "The Empty Hearse" (S3E1) Sherlock's parents make a brief cameo appearance, and when the main characters spend Christmas with them in "His Last Vow" (S3E3), they appear to be warm and affectionate people. Mr. Holmes clearly loves Mrs. Holmes, and the pair care about their children and enjoy lavish musicals and line dancing. There's certainly no indication that either of them ever did anything to traumatize their son. Of course, as Mr. and Mrs. Holmes are portrayed by Cumberbatch's real-life parents, Timothy Carlton and Wanda Ventham, it is not surprising that the pair are depicted warmly.

Though his parents appear to have done their best raising him, there are indications throughout the series that having an older brother who might also be on the spectrum may have affected Sherlock in various ways, and in the series' last episode to date, "The Final Problem," (S4E3), it is clear that the trauma inflicted by a psychotic sister has had a lasting effect on Sherlock's psyche. (The show strongly implies that Mr. and Mrs. Holmes are in no way responsible for their daughter's insanity, though Mycroft may have to shoulder some of the blame.) This backstory will be explored in another chapter, but

---

with them with reliable translations, so I am uncertain as to the status of their relationship with their daughter.

on *Sherlock*, this is a rare case of two caring parents who maintain a solid relationship with their child.

As for Takeuchi's *Miss Sherlock*, there is only one fleeting reference to the parents of Sherlock and Kento Futaba (Yukiyoshi Ozawa, who plays Sherlock's older brother, clearly a Japanization of Mycroft Holmes). In the first episode, Kimi Hatano (Ran Ito, playing the equivalent of Mrs. Hudson), says that she's happy to be Sherlock's landlady as she is deeply indebted to Sherlock's parents for unspecified services. They seem to have been kind to Hatano-sama, but otherwise no other information is provided about them, even whether they are alive or dead. Comparably, in *IQ 246*, the main character's father had a genius-level intellect, just like his son. Not much is told about their relationship, though Sharaku Homonji is clearly struggling under one aspect of the family legacy that has been placed upon him – the responsibility to marry and produce an heir. Otherwise, Homonji seems content to carry on the tradition of mental brilliance.

Moving on through a chronological study of these characters, *CSI*'s Grissom seems to have had a relatively happy childhood until he turned nine, when his father, a professor of science, passed away unexpectedly. In "Still Life" (S6E10), he recounts the story of his father's death, saying, "He came home from school, one hot humid day, and lay down on the couch. I was watching TV, my mom brought in some cold drinks, but she couldn't wake him up. No one would tell me why." This traumatic experience helped to fuel Grissom's interest in explaining causes of death. Later in life, his mother lost her hearing, which led to some added challenges, such as needing to learn sign language, but though this was an issue that needed to be addressed, it did not seem to strain their relationship, points addressed in the episode "Sounds of Silence" (S1E20).

Certainly death and hearing loss were not deliberate actions on the part of his parents, but they were understandably formative influences on Grissom.

Bobby Goren's tragic backstory is not revealed until midway through the show's run, and indeed, Goren is not even aware of the full extent of his family dysfunction until he uncovers it during an investigation in season six. Goren's family life was unhappy, as his father was unfaithful to his mother and irresponsible with the family finances, eventually abandoning his wife and family when Bobby was young, points referenced in "Blink" (S2E20) "The War at Home" (S6E6) and "Endgame" (S6E21). His mother battled mental illness for much of her life, further raising Goren's questions about his own stability.

Goren often wonders if his mental state will veer over the border between brilliance and madness, an anxiety that is provoked not solely by his mother's schizophrenia, but also by his older brother Frank (Tony Goldwyn), who has issues with both drug and gambling addictions. The former of which may be a form of self-medication for mental health issues inherited from his mother. The latter may have been picked up from his father's habits. Frank's combined problems mean that he is often forced to live on the streets, and Goren occasionally needs to extricate his brother from difficult situations, leading to strains in their relationship.

At the end of Season Six, "Endgame" (S6E21), the convicted murderer Mark Ford Brady (Roy Scheider) calls Goren with the goal of delaying his execution by potentially confessing to additional crimes. This leads Goren to dig into his family's history, leading him to realize that Brady was well-acquainted with Mrs. Goren. Upon questioning his mother, Goren learns that his own conception may have been the result of Brady raping Mrs. Goren, a point that is later confirmed by

DNA testing. Knowing that his own psyche is the combination of a serial killer and a schizophrenic, Goren grows increasingly uncertain of his long-term sanity, becoming occasionally erratic over the course of seasons seven and eight, culminating in his dismissal at the start of season nine before being rehired in season ten. After *Criminal Intent's* cancellation, on the *Law & Order: Special Victims Unit* episode "Acceptable Loss" (S14E4), Eames reveals that Goren is now off writing a book, and it's not clear whether he has permanently left or is simply on an extended sabbatical.

It is shown throughout the series that Monk has had OCD throughout his life, but it started to get out of control only after his wife's murder. That may have exacerbated the issue, but there are also indications that he had other significant trauma in his youth. There are a handful of brief references to Monk's childhood sprinkled throughout the series, but viewers see more details in the episode "Mr. Monk and Little Monk," (S4E8), and the collection of short episodes "Little Monk." In "Mr. Monk and Little Monk," Monk's mother (Rose Abdoo) is briefly depicted, as a woman uncomfortable with hugging. Though she's only on screen for a few seconds, her mannerisms suggest that she has many of the same tendencies that she passed on to her sons, and might have a form of OCD or autism herself. Certainly her unease with affection might be interpreted as coldness. There simply is not enough screen time to properly analyze her. She's rarely talked about, but in "Mr. Monk Goes Home Again" (S4E2), both Monk and his brother Ambrose (John Turturro) seem saddened when thinking of her, indicating that they have lasting affection for her.

Whatever issues Mrs. Monk might have had with emotions and touching, she stayed with her sons and raised them. Their father, Jack Monk, abandoned the family one night when he ostensibly went out for Chinese food, and they never saw him again until decades later. Like many of the detectives studied here, abandonment and maternal coldness are suggested as potential root causes for their social awkwardness, making it difficult to separate the psychological influence from the genetic impact.

Of all the characters studied here, perhaps none had a parent who embodied the "refrigerator mother" stereotype more than Dr. Martin Ellingham, and his father was no better. His relationship with his parents, Christopher (John Woodvine) and Margaret (Claire Bloom) is first introduced in "The Family Way" (S2E6). Neither is particularly warm to their son when they return after several years without speaking, and Christopher comes off as a selfish bully, denigrating his son for leaving a prominent medical career for a job as a small-town general practitioner, and attempting to compel his sister to sell the family farm. Margaret is comparably lacking in decency, and the coldness is so biting that Martin is left with no desire to repair their relationship. When Margaret returns in the sixth series after Christopher's death, she blames him for ruining her life with his existence. Martin's Aunt Ruth brings a psychological interpretation, arguing that his cold parents are responsible, at least in part, for his relationship troubles (S6E8, "Departure").

In the series finale, "Last Christmas in Portwenn," (S10E9), Margaret dies and Martin has memories of his unhappy childhood. Christmas was never a joyful time for him, as in one flashback scene, he comes downstairs to an empty house, as his parents preferred to celebrate their holiday without him, and his standard present each year was a pen and pencil set. A vision of Margaret in the finale has her berating and belittling him from beyond the grave, insisting that his personality is driving his family away from him. This leads Martin to make a conscious decision to make a grand gesture at Christmas, delighting his young son and bringing Martin's family closer together. Martin realizes that he can be a better parent than his own parents were, but it means adopting a more emotional and fun approach to his relationships.

On *Criminal Minds,* Spencer Reid had a difficult home life, due to his mother Diana's (Jane Lynch), long battle with the schizophrenia. Her frequent episodes of erratic behavior led to the breakup of his parents' marriage, and his father abandoned his wife and son. Diana's condition deteriorated, and when Reid came of age, he had her institutionalized for her own safety, though he felt guilty for the decision. Certainly his father walking out had psychological side-effects, and on multiple occasions he wonders if inherited mental illness will affect him at some point. But while his family experiences certainly were formative influences, they do not preclude autism, nor should they be construed as causes of pseudo-autistic behavior. It should be noted that many undiagnosed autistic people are frightened by their own mental states and reactions, and they wonder if they are developing a severe mental illness. Reid has more reason to fear for his mental state than most people due to his mental history, and certainly there is nothing to preclude having both autism and schizophrenia.

Viewers learn about Bones' backstory at the end of Season One, in "The Woman in Limbo" (S1E22). Her parents vanished when she was quite young, and her older brother Russ (Loren Dean) raised her for a while before turning her over to foster care. As a ward of the state, she endured numerous horrors, including cruel disciplinary measures. Once again, a double loss and traumatic upbringing were formative influences, which are not expressly credited as the cause of her autism-coded behavior, but are presented as factors in making her who she is. In "The Woman in Limbo," Bones examines the skeleton of a person who has been deceased for some time, and is blindsided by the discovery that the remains are her mother's. Over the course of the episode, she reunites with Russ and learns that her parents were actually fugitive criminals, and they abandoned their children in order to protect them from former colleagues who were pursuing them. Certainly all the years of not knowing her parents' fates took a toll on her, but in "The Girl in the Fridge" (S1E8), a prosecutor suggests that her seeming emotional detachment is a direct result of her parents vanishing without explanation. In that moment at least, the possibility that her demeanor is based on her innate brain chemistry is not considered.

    In another case of trauma being credited as the defining influence on a young psyche, over the course of the first season of *Dexter*, Dexter Morgan recovers the long-suppressed memory that when he was a very small child, his mother, a police informant who was helping to bring down a gang of drug dealers, was brutally murdered in a shipping container, and he and his older brother witnessed this vicious attack. The two boys were left in a pool of blood for an extended period before the police rescued them. This gory incident is credited with warping the minds of both boys, and instilling Dexter with an interest in the science of blood. While his mother appears to have been a loving single parent, Dexter's father was not in the picture while they were being raised, making no effort to connect with his son, though he did name Dexter his sole heir after his death. ("Father Knows Best," (S1E9)) From the end of the first season onwards, with his memories recovered, Dexter attributes all of his murderous urges – dubbed his "Dark Passenger"– to the bloody ordeal. And now that he has a cause, he simply accepts it and continues his stabbing ways more or less as he did before. No attempt is made to use this knowledge as a path to healing his damaged psyche. The Dark Passenger is treated as permanent and unconquerable until *New Blood*, when a strict routine helps suppress his murderous urges for many years.

L lost his parents at a very young age in an unspecified manner, and was raised in an orphanage. His mentor, Watari, served as his guardian and trained him to become a master detective. There is no explicit explanation in any of the versions of *Death Note* to explain exactly what made L what he is, but his parents' deaths may well have been one factor, as was Watari's education style, which was meant to generate astounding results from genius-level children. Mental or emotional strain caused by exposure to the horrific crimes L solved is also a possibility.

While in many cases the trauma these characters endured is briefly mentioned (often in a single episode, or a few small scenes), Lisbeth Salander's devastating backstory is a well-publicized part of her characterization, and is steadily revealed over the Swedish trilogy. Lisbeth's father was a criminal enjoying the protection of a branch of the Swedish government. He had no interest in being a father to his daughter, and was physically violent towards her mother. In an attempt to protect her mom, Lisbeth doused her father with accelerant and set him on fire. Though he survived, Lisbeth was institutionalized for the rest of her childhood and all of her adolescence, and a twisted doctor abused her while she was trapped in a mental hospital. Upon her release, she was placed under the care of a guardian. Her first guardian was a kindly fellow, but after a stroke incapacitated him, his replacement, Nils Bjurman, who controlled her money, raped her. As *The Girl Who Kicked the Hornet's Nest* illustrates, the situation was worsened by the fact that the authorities and other people who were supposed to be helping her ignored her pleas for help, and then turned the criminal justice system against her when she went outside the law to get revenge. Certainly these horrific experiences shaped many aspects of her personality and worldview, but a biological influence on her psyche is not suggested.

The backstory provided in *The Girl in the Spider's Web* is based on a continuation novel, and as it is David Lagercrantz's take on Steig Larsson's original characters, the new information added does not necessarily exist in the same universe as the narrative with the original trilogy. Certainly the Rapace and Mara iterations are not telling a story where a long-lost sister was a factor. The opening scene indicates that her father was sexually abusing both of his daughters, whereas before his cruelty was directed mainly towards Lisbeth's mother.

Abed never suffered traumas as severe as many of the characters discussed here, but he did endure emotional pain as a result of his parents' divorce. His parents broke up when he was a child, and Abed often wondered if his father blamed him for putting a strain on the marriage. Abed's father raised him, and by the time Abed went to college, his mother played an increasingly small role in his life, remarrying and enjoying a new family he'd never met, which had a crushing effect on Abed. The fact that his mother dedicated herself to her new family affected him deeply. ("Abed's Uncontrollable Christmas," S2E11)

Important details of Saga's backstory are revealed in the third season of *The Bridge*, as her mother arrives and chastises her for breaking up their family. Viewers learn that Saga believed her parents were abusing her and her sister Jennifer, with her mother Marie-Louise (Ann Petrén) poisoning them as a form of Munchausen by Proxy. Unable to prove the poisoning at that time, to save her sister, Saga falsely accused her parents of physical abuse and sent them to prison. Unfortunately, Saga could not repair the damage done to her sister's mental state, and her sister committed suicide. During the third season, Saga's mother confronts her, proclaiming her total innocence and saying that she needs to reconcile with her father before he dies. In addition, Marie-Louise attempts to convince Saga that her own emotional ineptitude led to Jennifer's suicide. When Marie-Louise dies soon after her husband, there are clues pointing towards murder, though Saga correctly deduces that her mother committed suicide and framed her. Saga is not able to convince the authorities of this, and winds up being wrongly convicted of her mother's murder soon after the events of Season Three. At the start of Season Four, Saga has managed to have the conviction overturned, and by the season's end, she has found proof that her mother did indeed sicken her daughters due to Munchausen by Proxy, and Jennifer's suicide was due to her mother's negative influence. Once again, the formative influence on a person with autism is shown to be horrific parenting.

In the American version, Sonya Cross was given a new backstory, consisting of a murdered sister and a still-alive but comatose killer, leaving Sonya with no answers as to why something so terrible happened to her sibling. Additionally, Sonya's mother Gail (Tamara Clatterbuck) is shown to have substance abuse and mental health problems, living on the streets. Gail appears briefly twice in the second season as a crabby "refrigerator," sniping at her daughter's actions and sartorial choices, and providing little compassion. Next to nothing is revealed about Sonya's father.

As for Elise in *The Tunnel*, her parents are not characters in *The Tunnel*, and few details are given about her upbringing.

Christopher Boone in *The Curious Incident of the Dog in the Night-Time* displayed autistic traits since he was very small, so the traumatic incidents that propel this action of the story clearly did not cause his condition. It is revealed throughout the play that the household was never happy. His parents' relationship was never strong, and even when his mother, Judy (Nicola Walker), is delighted to see him again, she can't help mentioning how Christopher's condition put a strain on their home life, placing herself in the role of the victim of an uncaring husband and a son who made life difficult for her. Christopher's father, Ed (Paul Ritter), is shown to have a violent temper, and when his mother left the family, Ed lied and told Christopher she was dead, keeping her letters from him. It is never revealed why Judy allowed two years to pass without attempting to visit or call her son, only that she decided that he was angry with her and chose to leave him alone until he was ready. She's certainly caring and protective towards her son when she sees him, though she points out how he broke some of her toes during one of his meltdowns. It is not clear exactly when that incident happened. Notably, she doesn't qualify that with an acknowledgment that it was an accident, and he wasn't aware of what he had done while he was having an episode. Ed is often protective of his son and wants him to succeed academically, but he also has verbal explosions, and like Judy, he often blames Christopher for responses that he cannot control.

On *Murdoch Mysteries,* Watts' parents both died when he was quite young. As a result, he was left with so few memories of them that he did not even realize until much later in life that his family was Jewish. He was left with his beloved older sister Clarissa (Elizabeth Whitmere), who disappeared suddenly, leaving him heartbroken. He was largely raised by a kind-hearted landlady who treated him like a son; as an adult, Watts was determined to track down his long-lost sister. When he finally found her in the episode "Hades Hath No Fury"

(S10E15), she turned out to be a "refrigerator sister," showing no warmth towards him. She abandoned him when he was twelve when she decided she didn't want to be tasked with raising him, and left him with no explanation, only anxiety and questions. She only confesses this after a previous lie that painted her as a victim – she has a habit of telling stories that make her look like a victim, and the men in her life appear controlling, and it is implied that she lies to make herself look like the victim. She tells Watts, "I left you because I did not wish to be chained into a life of servitude. I left you because I didn't want you. That's the truth." When she leaves for parts unknown, making it clear she has no interest in rebuilding her relationship with her brother, Watts is devastated, but the extent of the psychological and emotional damage is unclear. A colleague tells him, "You didn't choose your sister. In fairness, she didn't choose you." True enough, but in further fairness, Watts' sister did not choose to be honest with him earlier, sparing him a lifetime of worry.

Similarly, Murdoch's family was also broken, though in a different manner. His mother died when he was small, and for well into his adult life, he believed his father Harry (Stephen McHattie murdered her. In the show's first season (S1E6, "Let Loose the Dogs"), his father explains that her death was an accident and he had nothing to do with it, though as only Murdoch's father's word is given as evidence, there is no way to know for sure that Mrs. Murdoch's death was as innocent as he says. Murdoch's acceptance of this unverifiable tale seems uncharacteristic, though it's a special case, as it *is* his own father. Murdoch was raised in boarding schools, and he lost touch with his beloved sister, Susannah (Michelle Nolden), only meeting her again in adulthood, shortly before she died.

Holly Gibney's family background is one of the first details viewers learn about her in her first appearance in *Mr. Mercedes*. When Lupe's Holly enters the narrative midway through season one, she is clearly shaky and upset, having problems taking care of herself and interacting with others. At this point, she is living under the care of her parents, and her mother, Charlotte (Laila Robins) is a typical example of a "refrigerator mother." When Holly is in obvious distress, Charlotte is unsympathetic. She coldly rebukes Holly for her stimming and discomfort, treating her like a badly behaved child, and showing no compassion for what her daughter's going through at that moment. There is no attempt to understand what her daughter's thought processes are, no attempt to ameliorate her distress, only frosty reprimand. Once Holly receives her inheritance, thereby achieving independence, her parents vanish from the narrative, and they appear to have become peripheral to her life. Though they play no further role in the television series *Mr. Mercedes*, their fates are revealed in works written after the close of the Bill Hodges trilogy. By the novella *If It Bleeds*, Holly's father has died, and Charlotte loses some of her sharpness with his passing. In the novel *Holly*, King kills off Charlotte when Charlotte refused mask protocols and the vaccine during the pandemic.

Erivo's Holly's background has been substantially altered for *The Outsider*. Few details are given as to her early years, but there's a brief reference that her parents submitted her to a battery of tests in order to diagnose her mental state and "cure" it. In *The Outsider*, Holly's mother has passed away, and up until she died, she was caring for her daughter. No specifics are given as to the tenor of their relationship, and Holly is fully independent in this series, so it's unclear just how much care she needed from her mother. There is no indication of resentment from Erivo's Holly over her parents subjecting her to so much examination, though the tests do seem to have been somewhat traumatic.

Bart Bromley in *The Night Clerk* has one of the most caring and protective parents of the characters discussed in this study. He lives with his mother, Ethel (Helen Hunt), who cares deeply about him and gives him plenty of space. He rarely leaves the basement aside from work and errands, and Ethel uncomplainingly cooks his meals and leaves them at the top of the stairs, where he retrieves them soon after she leaves and eats them in solitude. Ethel is a widow. It is not made clear when her husband died, but it is stated that his passing had a devastating effect on Bart. Late in the movie, when he breaks his usual routine and eats with her, she says nothing but looks pleased. When the police suspect him of complicity in the crime, she defends her son fiercely and shields him from continued questioning. Ultimately, Ethel deeply loves her son and wants a closer relationship with him. Perhaps the only criticism one might direct towards her parenting is the fact that she gives him too much distance, and if she had supervised him more closely, she could have stopped him from recording other people.

Professor T has a classic example of a traumatizing childhood, and a continually strained maternal relationship. Throughout the first series, it's made clear that the professor's father was an angry and abusive man who also may have been an alcoholic. When he was a boy, Professor T wandered into the hall of the family home to find his father hanging from a noose. Subsequent episodes indicate that there was more to his father's death than a simple suicide, though as of the end of the second series, it's unclear whether some of the imagery consists of memories he's had access to all this time, whether these were repressed memories finally being remembered, or if these are fantasies.

Professor T's relationship with his mother can best be described as strained. Adelaide Tempest (Frances de la Tour) is an artist, as demonstrative as Jasper is restrained, and her displays of emotion and even her presence seem to aggravate Jasper and often send him into a panic. The first series does not delve into the root causes of their relationship, but the DVD special features indicate that there is genuine love between the two, though Adelaide seems to have a vested interest in keeping her son from exploring his own past. She's certainly not a refrigerator, but she's definitely hiding secrets from her son, and she tries to manipulate him on multiple occasions to behave as she prefers.

Woo Young-Woo grew up with a single father, who allowed her to believe that her mother had died in childbirth. This was a lie – her unmarried parents, Woo Gwang-ho (Jeon Bae-soo) and Tae Soo-mi (Jin Kyung) were classmates in law school and dating, and Tae Soo-mi became pregnant. Not wanting the stigma of a child born out of wedlock, Tae Soo-mi broke off the relationship and it's implied she was planning to end the pregnancy when Woo Gwang-ho tearfully begged her to have the baby, saying he'd raise the child himself, drop out of law school, and make sure that neither he or their daughter ever crossed Tae Soo-mi's path again. Tae Soo-mi eventually agreed, and Wo- Gwang-ho followed the deal. Tae Soo-mi eventually became one of the most respected lawyers in South Korea, was a candidate for an important government position, and presumably married before having a son who also had autism.

In flashback scenes, a sad Woo Young-woo sees intact families at school and asks her father why she does not have a mother. (S1E6. "If I Were a Whale"), Without Woo Gwang-ho realizing it, Woo Young-Woo got an answer to her question, one day when her grandmother was babysitting her, her grandmother had too much to drink and told her the whole story, though her mother's name wasn't mentioned. There's a hint that her grandmother resented Woo Young-woo for existing, as raising a special needs child derailed her son's career. Woo Young-Woo never spoke of this to her father, and only told him about this after he finally informed her that Tae Soo-mi was her mother. Once Tae Soo-mi learns of Woo Young-Woo's existence, she chooses not to try to build a relationship with her, and instead tries to get Woo Young-Woo and Woo Gwang-ho to move to the United States, so Woo Young-Woo's existence isn't discovered, leading to a scandal that could destroy her political ambitions.

If the viewer is uncharitably inclined, Tae Soo-mi might be viewed as a classic case of a "refrigerator mother," though she had no influence on her daughter during her developmental years. If one considers a more charitable interpretation of Tae Soo-mi's character, she may be seen as a woman driven to succeed in her chosen career, and possibly having a much milder case of autism than her children.

A critical consequence of these depictions of autistic characteristics in the media is that they can teach casual viewers that autism is something *inflicted* on some, not an *inherent* form of brain structure. Many people may watch these shows and conclude that autism in the result of someone doing something terrible to you. It is an even darker version of the "refrigerator mother" theory. In these dramatic portrayals, autism is the result of abuse or trauma. It leads viewers to wonder, even assume, that if someone is autistic, that something horrible happened to that person throughout that individual's formative years. That is an unfair assumption, and one which may need to be challenged in future depictions of characters with autism.

CHAPTER SIX
Wardrobe Functions

Though it is certainly not a characteristic unique to people with autism, many individuals on the spectrum are known for wearing distinctive clothing. There is a stereotype that people with autism may dress a trifle more eccentrically than the average person, but this is by no means universal. Many autistic people prefer to blend in and remain unnoticed. But in the film and TV productions discussed here, more than half of the potentially autistic sleuths demonstrate a distinctive style of dressing, often wearing exactly the same outfit (or at least, a notable piece of clothing) most of the time. More often than not, the clothes they wear reflect their characters.

Some of these characters have limited choice in what they wear, as their job requires a uniform. Male detectives on the official police force, for example, are expected to wear a suit and tie, and often regulations provide little room for individuality. In *Murdoch Mysteries*, the title character habitually wears a black suit and black Homburg hat, which is his signature item of clothing. Detective Watts demonstrates a bit more variety to his outfits, sometimes wearing a black suit with a gray vest, or a grey pinstriped suit, or more colorfully, a green checked suit, a color not worn by other detectives. Whatever suit he wears, it is always topped with a homburg hat like Murdoch's, only Watts' is gray with a black band.

Other characters regularly wear clothing similar to what thousands of other people wear on a daily basis. On *Bones*, Bones generally wears a blazer and blouse with jeans, or some variation of that outfit. Abed on *Community* tends to wear a t-shirt and an open sweatshirt or hoodie or button-down shirt with jeans. In the National Theatre Live production of *The Curious Incident of the Dog in the Night-Time*, Christopher wears a blue hoodie and tan pants, an outfit indistinguishable from those of other young men his age. He does voice one distinctive rule regarding his fashion sense, and that is due to his revulsion towards the color yellow.

But while some of these sleuths' clothing choices are extremely typical wardrobes today, many characters discussed here wear clothes that are distinctive, even iconic.

Perhaps the most iconic outfit connected to Sherlock Holmes is the deerstalker hat and Inverness cape, items that do not factor in the original stories, but made their way into the public consciousness through illustrations and their usage in stage and screen adaptations. As many devoted Holmesians know, under the standards of the time, Inverness capes and deerstalkers were strictly country wear, and were not worn on the streets of London. In the Downey *Sherlock Holmes*, the title character's regular wardrobe is not too different from that most of the other men, with no item particularly standing out in the wider public's imagination. Meanwhile, the title character in *Miss Sherlock* has a strong interest in fashion, and often upbraids Wato for being insufficiently stylish. While several items of Sherlock's wardrobe are worn on multiple occasions, like a knee-length brown coat or a black leather jacket, there's no real stand-out article.

It is Benedict Cumberbatch's wardrobe on *Sherlock* that is distinctive, particularly his outerwear. On *Sherlock*, the title character's full-length Belstaff coat has become a popular culture icon of its own. Dark gray and made of wool tweed, the style is descended from the greatcoats of the early twentieth century. Often worn with a blue-grey scarf and covering upscale dress shirts and suits (though worn without a tie), the coat has become so linked to the character that it's notable that none of the episodes of *Sherlock* are set during the hot summer months.

Certainly there's a dramatic element to the coat, as it's often filmed billowing behind him as he's running, creating the image of a superhero's cape. Certainly it's not more functional than any other item of clothing, and it is sufficiently distinctive that it actually serves as a bit of a hindrance on the many occasions when Sherlock's trying to track a suspect, as it is a conspicuous item. There seems to be a deep emotional attachment between the garment and its wearer, as when Sherlock returns from the "dead" at the start of Series Three, he dons his coat as if he's stepping back into his own skin. It should be noted that he does not need to use the coat as a security blanket, as he's perfectly capable of going out without it. When he's called to Buckingham Palace in "A Scandal in Belgravia," he's content to wear nothing at all except a bedsheet, mostly for the purpose of thumbing his nose at the people who dragged him out from 221B.

  An in-joke of the series is that Sherlock is often compelled to wear a deerstalker cap against his personal preference. Originally snatched up to cover his face from paparazzi, a viral photograph of him wearing it causes it to be inextricably linked with his popular image, even more so than his coat. By the fourth series episode "The Lying Detective" (S4E2), a room full of children at a hospital seem to wish he'd worn the hat to visit them, and at the end of the episode, he dons it of his own volition for a public appearance, though he seems to take no pleasure in wearing it, noting that the headgear has in effect become part of his brand. It is a moment where he grudgingly accepts his own iconography.

  Monk has one of the most consistent sartorial styles discussed here. Aside from when he goes undercover, he always wears the same outfit, a brown suit, brown loafers, and a light-colored dress shirt buttoned up to the top, but no tie. He not only has many identical items, but as viewers learn in "Mr. Monk Goes to a Fashion Show (S4E10)," he also insists that all of his shirts be approved by the same garment inspector, Number 8. This reflects his OCD tendencies and his love of stability, and it is notable that in the series finale, once he has achieved a level of happiness he had long ago given up on achieving, he adopts a slightly more casual version of his standard wardrobe, though he returns to his traditional outfit once he enters a darker post-pandemic mental state in the follow-up movie *Mr. Monk's Last Case*.

Though most of the time Dexter wears non-distinctive clothes that are appropriate for the Miami heat, there is one time when, given the choice, he almost invariably wears the same outfit: when he is about to kill one of his targets. Having performed his standard ritual of drugging and immobilizing a target, leaving the soon-to-be victim pinned to a table with tape and plastic wrap in a plastic-draped room, Dexter dons a brown Henley shirt and tan cargo pants. No specific backstory or reason for this wardrobe choice is ever given, it simply is the self-imposed wardrobe he wears when he commits a murder. There may be some practical issues – the cargo pants may hold various tools, and as on numerous occasions his shirt gets splattered with blood, sometimes heavily, the wide-open neck of the Henley shirt makes it easier to remove without blood getting in his hair, though a button-down shirt would pose even less risk of smearing gore on his face and hair. One point is never made clear on the show – when does Dexter clean his bloodstained clothes? He's almost never shown changing into or out of his "kill outfit," and bloodstains are notoriously difficult to remove. During Season Four, he can't use his own house's clothes washer due to the presence of his family. One wonders if he simply disposes of the ruined clothing and buys multiple versions of the same garments, but there's no indication that he tosses the stained items into the ocean or otherwise destroys them.

L always wears the same outfit in the anime series: a white long-sleeved t-shirt and blue jeans, and he goes barefoot wherever possible. It reflects his lack of interest in formality and fashion, especially when compared to the suited professional policemen. Casual clothes also allow him greater flexibility for sitting in his preferred crouching position, though he does not swap out his jeans for athletic pants when playing tennis.

When L gives a speech at a large college orientation ceremony after achieving perfect scores on all of the entrance exams, several of the attendees comment on his appearance, saying that he must be some sort of mad genius in order to dress like that. Whether L is aware of people's reactions and assumptions of him based on his wardrobe is unknown.

The live-action television series adjusts L's outfit as well as his personality. Instead of a long-sleeved T-shirt, he wears a white button-down shirt, and every time he notices a spot or some fraying, he asks Watari for a replacement shirt, often leading to a mild venting of disgust from Watari about L's "willful requests." Instead of blue jeans, this version of L wears white pants. Notably, some of the Asian productions of the musical version have L adopting the all-white look, but in the filmed production, L wears what he does in the anime version, although in a couple of scenes he wears an olive-green jacket that is nowhere to be found in the anime. In the Netflix movie, L wears mostly black, including a hoodie and mask, which serve the functional purpose of protecting his anonymity.

While in many cases, the wardrobe choices of the characters discussed here inadvertently or unconsciously set them apart from other people, in Lisbeth Salander's case, there is a level of *deliberate* distinction in her choice of appearance. Not only does she almost exclusively wear black, but her hair is dyed black, and she has multiple piercings and body art, all as part of a punk-Goth look.[2] In *The Girl With the Dragon Tattoo* (Swedish version) and *The Girl in the Spider's Web*, Lisbeth is told on a couple of occasions that she has made herself ugly, though in both cases the person who denigrates her appearance is a villain. Certainly her look gets attention, and in every movie, characters respond with looks of shock, confusion, and even disgust when they see her. Invariably, Lisbeth herself never shows any signs of caring what people think of her, though she also (at least not in the films) never discussions her reasons for adopting the appearance she has.

In *The Girl Who Kicked the Hornet's Nest*, there's a level of defiance as well, when Lisbeth is on trial, and might wind up in prison or a mental hospital for the rest of her life. Under traditional courtroom strategies, Lisbeth ought to adopt a more conservative look for the duration of the legal proceedings, as a conventional appearance might be likelier to impress the judges favorably. Instead, she wears her normal clothing, keeps her body modifications on full display, and styles her hair into a mohawk. It is an act of defiance, showing that she does not intend to change her personal style for any reason and that she does not intend to kowtow to any potential prejudices of the judiciary regarding her appearance, even if her entire future is on the line. The exception is when she needs to disguise herself

---

[2] Though on *24*, Chloe O'Brian's clothes are fairly conventional, in her final appearance to date in *24: Live Another Day*, she adopts a look very similar to Lisbeth, as she has left her government counterterrorism job after being arrested for assisting Jack Bauer in fleeing the authorities, and now (wrongly) blames the government for the deaths of her husband and son. As she is now working for a group striving to expose government malfeasance, it's possible that her makeover is a direct reference to Lisbeth Salander.

for undercover work, where she uncomplainingly dons a wig and less conspicuous clothing, and removes her piercings. It emphases a level of control, when she has often lacked power in her personal life, and it also demonstrates the level of contempt she has for the court, as her previous conviction and legal guardianship were the result of pressure from sinister forces with the power to sway Sweden's institutions. By dressing as she does, Lisbeth thumbs her nose at a legal system that has been corrupted and has wronged her in the past.

In some ways, this raises the question of authenticity. Does Lisbeth dress the way she does because she inherently likes it, or does she like how it causes other people to respond? Or is could be a bit of both? That is an unanswered question that is open to interpretation, but in the cases of other characters studied here, they clearly choose their clothing because it literally suits them, not because of what other people think.

One of Saga's trademark characteristics is that she always wears the same outfit, consisting of a long brown military greatcoat over a brown leather jacket and a grey sweater, and dark leather pants. On occasion she changes into a dark blue T-shirt, but that is the extent of her wardrobe. The only time she's seen wearing anything different is when she has been wrongly imprisoned at the start of season four, and wears a pale prison sweat suit. Upon her release, when she changes into her iconic outfit, the scene is framed as if to show that she's becoming herself again and reclaiming her own identity. While Saga's long coat and leather pants serve a functional purpose in protecting her from the Scandinavian cold (though it is unclear how much the weather affects her, as she never wears a hat), no reason is given as to why she has selected these pieces as her daily wear. No backstory or reasons for liking these garments are provided.

In contrast, Sonya's signature piece of clothing in the American version has a clearly outlined emotional connection, and she wears it regularly despite its impracticality. Sonya wears a faded tan leather motorcycle jacket most of the time, and interestingly, the entire jacket is not shown all at once. Throughout the first season, different closeups and perspectives of the jacket are shown sporadically, providing more information at different times. The jacket is not solid leather, as patches around the shoulders are leopard print fabrics, there's a sketch of a horse across the back and a patch of a tiger at the bottom of the front, safety pins are clipped in a line on one shoulder, another sketch of a tiger is on a more unobtrusive fold of the leather, a red star has been drawn on one arm, a line of little arrows runs along another sleeve, the right cuff has been repaired with duct tape, and the coloring of the battered leather varies widely.

It is revealed midway through the first season that the leather jacket initially belonged to her older sister, Lisa, and after Lisa was murdered, Sonya began wearing it. Clearly the jacket is a connection to her sister. Though Lisa's killer is known, his motive for the crime is not, as Sonya's mentor, Hank, when confronting the murderer, shot him and left him permanently unconscious and unresponsive, so Sonya has no answer to the "why" for the crime, and she often puzzles over this in her spare time Sonya's gruff, unsympathetic mother disapproves of her wearing the jacket, saying that the garment does not fit her. (Though it is not tailored to her figure, the jacket does fit her pretty well.)

While the emotional connection to the jacket is not and does not need to be spelled out on the show, it is notable that Sonya never shows discomfort wearing it in the sweltering sun of Texas and Mexico. The rest of her wardrobe is far less distinctive– she wears widely varying shirts; mostly white, black, and gray; and black pants or jeans.

Notably, on *The Tunnel*, Elise's clothing is much like everybody else's. There's nothing particularly unique or eye-catching about it. While leather is an integral part of Saga and Sonya's wardrobe, Elise briefly wears a black leather jacket in the first season, but it soon disappears, and it's not part of the character's signature look as such items are in the other versions of *The Bridge*. Elise essentially dresses just like everybody else.

On *Chasing Shadows*, Sean wears a suit like most detectives, and a dark blue coat that extends a bit below his waist. There's nothing especially distinctive about the coat, and there doesn't seem to be any backstory behind it, but at one point, when visiting a facility, he is asked to remove it temporarily, and he seems to express some discontent with that. Perhaps he is more comfortable wearing it, but his connection to the coat is not explored aside from that moment.

On *Professor T*, the title character is almost always seen wearing an immaculate three-piece suit and tie. It demonstrates his formality, his attention to detail, and reflects the rigidity of his behaviors. Indeed, the stiffness of his regular wardrobe is so fitting for his character that it seems somehow wrong when he wears anything else. In the first series' third episode, "Tiger Tiger," the Professor is badly shaken by a traumatizing flashback inspired by his mother's presence, and after he falls down the stairs, he's taken to the hospital for treatment for his injured leg. As the trousers of his suit needed to be cut away by the doctor, for most of the episode he is compelled to wear a tracksuit, chosen because it was the only item at the hospital gift shop in his size. The incongruity of the outfit is noted by his peers, and at the episode's end, his mother waspishly comments that he can't pull off the "casual wear" look. In S2E2, "The

Mask Murders," Professor Tempest is hospitalized for appendicitis, and surrounded by all of the potential sources of infection that can be found in a hospital, he's on edge and curt towards his nurse. It's only when he receives some of the comforts of home that he's able to regain his focus on the case. Jettisoning the hospital garb in favor of his own dressing-gown does wonders to alleviate his stress and return his mind to its usual level of acuity.

Doc Martin, similarly, always wears a two-piece dark blue suit and a tie, representing his personal formality, almost never wearing anything else except at bedtime.

Of the characters discussed here, Woo Young-Woo is the only one who states that the fashion choices she makes are connected to her autism. While most of the other lawyers at her firm wear dark professional suits, Woo Young-Woo chooses soft fabrics that do not aggravate her sensory issues. In the first episode, which bears the same name as the series, her father helps her with her new outfit, assuring her that he has cut away all the tags, presumably because the sensation of them rubbing against her neck is unpleasant to her. She usually wears a jacket or sweater made of her preferred materials, often cut more loosely than the clothes of her female peers for added comfort. She almost invariably wears skirts to work as well, and is rarely shown wearing pants, except pajama bottoms when she sleeps, or jeans in flashbacks of her as a small child, most likely before she was diagnosed and was able to verbalize her sensory issues with fabric texture. As the style of her clothes causes her to stand out from her peers at the law firm, the other lawyers often look at her distinctive clothing, but little is ever said to her face. No one suggests that she adopt a more conventional business professional wardrobe, and it seems to be silently understood that her clothes are chosen to help her function better.

Clothing and fashion choices reflect individual personality, and distinctive choices are certainly not limited to people with autism. But by illustrating the wide variety of sartorial choices these characters make, it illustrates the diversity of the autistic experience, stressing how autism is not a homogenous condition.

CHAPTER SEVEN
Visual Representations of Mental Processes and Observation

Sometimes the medium of film doesn't capture the entirety of reality. No camera can fully portray the complexity of the workings of the human mind. As such, artistic license needs to be taken in order to recreate mental processes. Stylized or surrealistic imagery is used in order to replicate the thinking and reacting of people with autism.

The visual depictions of how the autistic organize their thoughts and react to the world around them are naturally not representative of how the entirety of the autistic population thinks. There is no uniformity in how the autistic think. When dramatic productions use visual imagery to illustrate the mind of an autistic character, the results do not reflect all or even the majority of how certain people with autism mentally process information. I can state, however, when I first watched the Downey *Sherlock Holmes*, the Cumberbatch *Sherlock*, and the filmed stage production of *The Curious Incident of the Dog in the Night-Time*, I was stunned, because for the first time I saw the visual processes of my mind portrayed on the screen, and at the time, I did not know of anyone else on earth whose brains reacted to information in the same way that I do.

One of the first scenes in the 2009 movie *Sherlock Holmes* that strongly reflects how a person with autism might respond in a busy social situation takes place in a crowded restaurant, where Holmes meets Watson's (Jude Law) fiancée Mary Morstan (Kelly Reilly). As he waits for his dining companions, Holmes fidgets in his chair, his eyes darting around the room, registering little sights and sounds in the cacophony of diners around him, growing steadily more unsettled until the others finally arrive.

Arguably the stylistic hallmark of the Downey movies is the depiction of Holmes thinking out every action and potential consequence before carrying out those actions, with the predicted events playing out in his mind, and the actual results matching with remarkable similarity. The first example of this is when Holmes is boxing, plans a strategy to take down an aggressive opponent. When Holmes tries to forfeit the match in order to track down Irene Adler, his opponent spits at his head. In response, Holmes thinks, "This mustn't register on an emotional level." He then considers a series of actions to defeat the other boxer, including distraction through throwing a handkerchief, blocking the anticipated punches, discombobulating his opponent with blows to the ears, and a series of punches and kicks in sensitive areas to finish the job, mentally concluding, "In summary: ears ringing, jaw fractured; three ribs cracked, four broken; diaphragm hemorrhaging. Physical recovery: six weeks. Full psychological recovery: six months. Capacity to spit at back of head... neutralized." Holmes carries out his plan, and it all works out in Holmes' favor.

It is worth noting that his attack on McMurdo doesn't go exactly as planned, and that the elbow block maneuver has to be changed when McMurdo's post-discombobulated attack does not follow the precise course that Holmes initially anticipates. This illustrates that Holmes is neither psychic nor rigidly stuck in his planned actions. Should the circumstances warrant it, Holmes can change his tactics at an instant's notice to something more effective. This scene does indicate a level of flexibility that many people with autism do not always enjoy as sometimes any deviation from a planned course of action can lead to less than ideal reactions. Certainly strong internal responses, like an autistic meltdown, cannot always be quelled by calmly telling oneself, "This mustn't register on an emotional level." But the long-term planning and detached calculations can often reflect the approach people with autism take towards their future actions, often visualizing them in intense detail. This is a form of rehearsal that can prove helpful.

    Of course, planning actions and reactions prior to their occurrence is not limited solely to the autistic. At the climax of *Sherlock Holmes: A Game of Shadows*, Holmes confronts Moriarty (Jared Harris) after impoverishing the latter's criminal network, and it soon becomes clear that the next clash between the two will be physical, not purely mental. Holmes performs his trademark mental predictions and plans, but soon after beginning, Moriarty unsettles him with the unspoken line, "Come now, you really think you're the only one who can play this game?" Much like in the aforementioned scene, both men predict how the other will respond physically, and respond with counter-moves. Due to Holmes' injury, Moriarty is convinced that his victory is preordained, but Holmes defeats the Professor through an unexpected maneuver – a quick distraction with some blown pipe ashes, and pulling Moriarty with him over the wall and into Reichenbach Falls.

    In another Sherlock Holmes franchise, the Cumberbatch Sherlock's mental processes are portrayed on-screen through words and less frequently images floating in the air. When he looks at a person or object, words appear on-screen, indicating the deductions he has inferred through his observations. At times, memories and clues float through the air, and he can move them around by swiping them with his hands, much like one might with a tablet screen. Sherlock's use of the phrase "memory palace" is a term for mentally organizing information that has been used for centuries, as people can better access large quantities of information by organizing it into imaginary rooms in their minds.

In *IQ 246: The Cases of a Royal Genius*, in nearly every episode, Sharaku Homonji's mental processes are represented visually and audibly in a meditation scene. Shortly before the episode's climax, Homonji retreats to his private study, where he sits at a table and plays a game of Go with himself as important clues from previous lines of dialogue are heard. The recurring scene illustrates how Homonji's brain processes information, and organizes disarray. Chess-playing is a frequent theme in Holmes adaptations, such as in the Downey *A Game of Shadows*, where it symbolizes the mental duel between Holmes and an opponent. In this Nipponized version of the Holmes mythos, the ancient Asian board game is a form of meditation, and this solitaire version of the game, whether it is seen as a puzzle or a complex equation to be solved, serves as a visual representation of how Homonji's mind seeks out elegant solutions in a systematic manner.

It is not just iterations of Sherlock Holmes that have tried to portray different ways of mentally processing information on-screen. Once again, the purpose of these essays is not to prove that the characters discussed here officially have autism. To reiterate, the goal of these essays *is to use the characterizations in the analyzed productions in order to provide a resource for people with autism to explain their condition to others.*

At times, when we see into the mind of a detective, it is simply to see reenactments of the crimes. Sporadically on *Murdoch Mysteries*, viewers see the title character play out situations in his mind as he attempts to recreate the crime. It's a dramatic technique that's used on many crime dramas, and there's nothing distinctly autistic about it, although it does show Murdoch's logical and orderly mindset.

Comparably, Will Graham's mental processes are often shown recreating crimes, as all he needs to do is study a crime scene, and he can mentally recreate what happened with uncanny accuracy. Upon observing a scene, he can unwind time in his imagination, and place himself in the killer's shoes, going through every violent action, and saying "this is my design" to accentuate when the murderers do something distinctively shaped against their own personalities. On a couple of occasions, we see depictions of hallucinations or imaginary images, sometimes influenced by Graham's first-season battle with encephalitis. When Will Graham hallucinates about a dark, monstrous wendigo or a stag creature, it represents the dark influence Hannibal Lecter is having on his psyche.

On occasion, Professor T mentally pictures an unusual scene to represent a thought going through his head. In "A Fish Called Walter" (S1E2), he awkwardly broaches a question to a suspect about her husband's alleged cheating. He handles the matter very indelicately, and the blatant nature of it all of it is reflected in his sudden realistic daydream, where a line of cheerleaders dances into the hall and does a routine, shouting out "ADULTERY!" Other hallucinations include seeing his mother's face everywhere during times of stress, reflecting the strained nature of their relationship, and he expresses his complex emotions over his lost love through imagining romantic scenes of dancing on rooftops.

Notably, both of the filmed staged productions use go beyond realism in order to replicate the autistic sleuth's mind processes. In *The Curious Incident of the Dog in the Night-Time*, lights, sounds, and props are used in order to demonstrate Christopher Boone's mental state, as heightened noises and flashing lights can demonstrate his growing overstimulation, and words, numbers, and pictures, often far too much for the audience to read in full, are projected upon the stage to show what's going through Christopher's head. Likewise, in the filmed musical version of *Death Note*, a couple of scenes with L show flashing screens displaying information connected to the case, such as in the song "The Game Begins," where L sings about his investigative process.

While the Swedish version of the Millennium trilogy is filmed realistically, both of the English-language versions of the Salander movies feature a CGI opening credits title sequence. David Fincher suggested that this sequence in *The Girl with the Dragon Tattoo* was meant to represent the unsettling dreams that Salander has throughout the series, often the result of her personal traumas. The nightmarish images of oily faces, technology coming to life in monstrous form, fire, and humans enduring violence and torture reflect the horrors Salander survived in her youth and formed her adult psyche. Though the surrealistic imagery is not exclusive to an autistic mindset, it does reflect how actual events can be mentally processed into larger-than-life forms.

A significant number of scenes in *Dexter* feature images from Dexter's imagination. Dexter's adoptive father Harry appears in flashbacks during the first two seasons, but from seasons three to eight, Harry is a consciously created product of Dexter's mind, and the two often discuss his crimes and how he plans to escape his opponents, both criminals and the official police. In these imaginary conversations, Dexter uses Harry as a sounding board for ideas and venting frustration, using his late parent as a collaborator in his murderers. In contrast, in *Dexter: New Blood*, Dexter's now-deceased sister Debra plays a similar role as an imaginary companion, only as his new life becomes increasingly more violent, she challenges his decisions and often serves as a conscience figure for him as a way that Harry never did. These conversations are important, not because of how the images are portrayed on the screen, but because of what they illustrate about Dexter's personal thoughts. The only other major look into Dexter's mind is his daydream at the end of season one, where he imagines a throng of people cheering him for the good he does for society with his killings.

In addition, during the sixth season, Dexter has two brief sexual encounters, the first with a former classmate who seduces him in an empty classroom at a high school reunion, and then again with a convenience store attendant he just met moments earlier. These interludes initially come across as real occurrences to the viewers, and Dexter never questions their veracity, but something does not gel about them. The scenes may reflect Dexter's increasing interest in sex, but the ideas of two attractive women wanting a quick, strings-free fling with Dexter in a public place seems more like fantasy than reality. The earlier case in particular has all the hallmarks of a revisited adolescent dream. Coupled with the fact that a major plot point in season six involves a character's inability to separate imagination from reality, these affairs may well be purely the result of Dexter's overactive imagination, allowing him to picture himself as a desirable man who can enjoy casual sex with none of the burden of an actual relationship, especially due to the fact that his three previous relationships caused him so much stress and devastating heartbreak. There's a bit of an ego trip in these scenes as well, as one woman claims to have spent two decades contemplating having sex with him, and the other is willing to become intimate with him after a minute's acquaintance and knowing nothing about him.

On *Extraordinary Attorney Woo*, Woo Young-Woo's mental processes are represented through CGI animation. At one point, Woo Young-Woo visualizes legal information as a series of floating rectangular screens, which she can swipe and move around like windows on an electronic tablet. Most notably, Woo Young-Woo visualizes a whale swimming through the air right before she has an intellectual epiphany that helps her either realize the truth behind a case or determine a strategy for winning in court. Her intense interest in whales represents the feelings of exhilaration she gets as she uses her extensive legal knowledge to make discoveries that her peers overlook; and the whales she imagines, with calm, rhythmic movements, have a soothing effect on her in potentially overwhelming situations.

Not all depictions of atypical minds are visual. In *The Outsider* episode "Dark Uncle" (S1E3), in response to Ralph Anderson's (Ben Mendelsohn) declaration that he has "no tolerance for the unexplainable" after Erivo's Holly Gibney qualifies the possibility of doppelgängers being a myth with an "if," Holly replies,

"Well then, sir, you'll have no tolerance for me… I can tell you what day May 1st lands on 204 years from now faster than any computer on Earth. I can look at a skyscraper for two seconds from a speeding car and tell you within six inches how tall that building is. And I can not only recite the lyrics of every rock and roll song written from 1954 to the present day, but I can tell you what Billboard chart position they were in week to week before they fell off completely. But you know what? I don't listen to music, because I don't like it. Heights make me throw up. And if you ask me what date it is today, I have to look at a calendar… When I was four years old, my parents took me to see a psychiatrist to be examined. That was what got the ball rolling. And, well, by the time I was eight years old, I had been tested, uh, studied, written about and videoed by psychiatrists, behaviorists, neuroscientists, and six different kinds of interdisciplinary socio-biologists. And you know what they said? 'F*** if I know.' So, Mr. Anderson, if I feel like using the conditional 'if,' then 'if's' the word, mockingbird."

When Ralph expresses shock that the Gibneys allowed their daughter to be tested like that, Holly replies, "They were scared. They thought the white coats could cure me." To which Ralph responds, "Cure you of being yourself?" It's a question Holly can't or won't answer, as after a brief moment of reflecting on it, she's compelled to leave the bar where they're conversing and recover her thoughts in solitude. This verbal description of her abilities illustrates how Erivo's Holly's brain can store information and assess her surroundings, and it also stresses that modern science is woefully inadequate at explaining how she is able to function as she is and why she was born with the brain she has. Ralph's point about how Holly's mind is who she is illustrates a paradigm shift. People with autism often think that there's something wrong with them before– and often after – their diagnosis. The possibility that there is nothing inherently wrong that needs correction with them can be more of a confounding shock than a relief.

In various forums, autistic people have complained about the "realism" of these depictions. Certainly there can be atypicality amongst the atypical, and all of these characters can arguably described as "eccentric savants" and many people with autism don't process information or respond to stimuli in the same way that others do. But as non-universal as these productions are, they have helped me immeasurably with communicating my thought processes to others. I compare this to several medicines. There are some medicines that help the afflicted enormously, but the same medication may affect other people with the same conditions adversely, with potentially serious side effects. (Personally, I have had horrifically negative reactions to every medication that is designed to affect brain function.) In many ways, these dramatic productions are similar. They are critical to my ability to connect to other people as a means of self-description. But I also understand that they are useless to others on the autism spectrum. Nevertheless, stylized depictions of the thought processes of people with autism can serve as a starting point for personal explanations of mental reactions.

In many of these visual representations, there is also an implication that the "incoming" sensations are connected to difficulties connecting with other people. If one's brain is juggling all of this, how can it manage anything else? What some of the other characters view as self-absorption or cluelessness is actually an attempt at holding oneself together, not to block out others. In many of these cases, the autistic character mentally withdraws from the social situation briefly, taking an opportunity to think and to organize responses. The creative depictions used here are metaphorical for some real-life people with autism, though in my case, some of these depictions, mainly those in the Sherlock Holmes adaptations, *The Curious Incident of the Dog in the Night-Time*, and *Extraordinary Attorney Woo* closely mirror my own thinking processes.

CHAPTER EIGHT
Love, Sex, and Autism

The course of true love never did run smooth, and for people on the autism spectrum, it often comes with more difficulties than it does for the neurotypical. Certainly rocky relationships are a hallmark of drama, but as portrayed in these productions, autism brings unique challenges for those involved. While the exact statistics are open to scrutiny, it is widely believed that the percentage of people with autism who are married or in a relationship is significantly below those of the general population. While the entertainment industry's portrayals of romance rarely replicate real life, in most cases, characters on the spectrum are often given extra hurdles to finding love.

Sleuths on the spectrum can be categorized into several categories, usually divided upon gender lines. Several of the characters discussed here wind up in happy relationships, though they can only find a fulfilling relationship through a particularly understanding and supportive partner. Many of the men are single and seem disinterested in relationships, sometimes almost to the point of asexuality or frigidity. In some cases, those who try to find a romantic partner proceed so awkwardly that their attempts at finding love are doomed to failure. These characters often would like a partner, but for multiple reasons, often connected to their personal mental states, cannot find or keep one. With very few exceptions, the autistic males who do find love are monogamous, essentially mating for life. As for the women, they tend to be divided into two basic categories. There are the naïve, inexperienced autistic women who need assistance navigating through the dating world, and who attract men who are intrigued by their seeming innocence, genuineness, and uniqueness. In contrast, other autistic women are portrayed as active and unrestrained sexually, indulging in affairs solely for physical gratification and with seemingly negligible emotional involvement, at least at first.

While once again, autistic traits are played up in contemporary adaptations of Sherlock Holmes to an extent that they would never have been considered in the original stories, there is plenty of material in the Holmesian Canon to paint the great detective as adverse to romance, preferring a life of cold intellectual pursuits instead of romantic entanglements. Though many readers wonder about his feelings for Irene Adler in "A Scandal in Bohemia," there is no proof of any actual relationship between them in the original Doyle stories. In the opening paragraph of the original short story "A Scandal in Bohemia," Watson writes that,

> *"It was not that he felt any emotion akin to love for Irene Adler. All emotions, and that one particularly, were abhorrent to his cold, precise but admirably balanced mind. He was, I take it, the most perfect reasoning and observing machine that the world has seen, but as a lover he would have placed himself in a false position. He never spoke of the softer passions, save with a gibe and a sneer. They were admirable things for the observer– excellent for drawing the veil from men's motives and actions. But for the trained reasoner to admit such intrusions into his own delicate and finely adjusted temperament was to introduce a distracting factor which might throw a doubt upon all his mental results. Grit in a sensitive instrument,*

or a crack in one of his own high-power lenses, would not be more disturbing than a strong emotion in a nature such as his."

Of course, many later writers have been unable to resist exploring Holmes' heart. The Downey Holmes has an on-again, off-again, romantically antagonistic relationship with Irene Adler (Rachel McAdams), and a fleeting line in the first movie implies that their romance was at one point physical in nature. A quip from Law's Watson indicates that Adler is the sole woman who has ever interested him romantically. The pair spar, flirt, and banter throughout the first film, with one initially coming out on top, then the other, and the relationship continues in a similar vein in the first act of the sequel, only to end when Holmes is left stunned by Adler's apparent death at the hands of Moriarty.

As the creators of *Sherlock* often take a meta approach to their subject matter Cumberbatch's Holmes addresses many of the questions readers have had about Holmes for decades. Starting in "A Scandal in Belgravia" (S2E1), Sherlock has an unconventional relationship with Irene Adler (Lara Pulver), who is reimagined in this series as a dominatrix with lesbian inclinations. On multiple occasions, she flirts with Sherlock, though it's up to interpretation how much of her interest in Holmes is genuine and how much is an attempt to manipulate him. After he saves her life, she texts him on occasion, though Sherlock later tells John in "The Lying Detective" (S4E2) he doesn't text back. Holmes' own feelings are hard to pin down, as he often seems confused by Adler's advances, and his opinion of Adler is ambiguous. For his part, John encourages Sherlock to attempt a relationship with Adler, though John is personally grieving the loss of his wife in "The Lying Detective," so his personal bereavement may be fueling his encouragement.

Sherlock never talks about his feelings for Irene, so the extent of his emotions towards her are open to interpretation. As his reaction to her cameo appearance in Sherlock's "mind palace" in "The Sign of Three" (S3E2) indicates, she enters his thoughts even when he doesn't want her to, but is it attraction? An appreciation for her mental challenge? A blow to his ego over the fact that she came within an inch of besting him in a duel of wits? Viewers can think as they choose, and whether Cumberbatch's Sherlock sees her as a potential love interest, an opponent, or something else depends on what the audience wants to see. For Irene's part, whether her texts have genuine affection for Sherlock in them, or whether they're a mind game power play, or if they're simply teasing Sherlock is similarly up for debate.

Given the level of distrust, gamesmanship, and manipulation between the two in both the Downey/McAdams and the Cumberbatch/Pulver takes on the Holmes/Adler connection, neither can be called a wholly healthy relationship, as love, attraction, and mutual respect are overshadowed by competition, suspicions of manipulation, and scorekeeping. Certainly there are worse bases for relationships, but at the heart of the problems in both cases (aside from Adler's criminal tendencies) is Holmes's work-focused mindset, which compels him to see Adler as either an opponent to be checkmated or an enigma to be solved.

Aside from Irene Adler, Cumberbatch's Sherlock has a few other potential love interests over the course of the series. Molly Hooper (Louise Brealey), the morgue employee with an obvious crush on Sherlock, would certainly date Sherlock if he ever asked her out, but he never makes a move, using her primarily as a source of assistance during his investigations. Over the course of the series, she has two failed relationships, the first being where Moriarty (Andrew Scott) dates her as part of a fiendish plan, the second being a brief engagement to a man with a close physical resemblance to Sherlock but none of his intelligence. It is unclear whether his similar sartorial choices to Sherlock's are his own preferences or if Molly selected his clothes for him. Sherlock's rejection of Molly is less based on her as it is his absorption in his work. He often treats her brusquely and thoughtlessly, particularly in the earlier seasons, but as part of his developing awareness of how his words and actions affect others, he steadily realizes that he does have feelings for her by "The Final Problem" (S4E3), though again, it's vague as to whether he simply feels fond friendship or actual amorous intent.

Notably, there are different levels of inequality on the Sherlock/Molly relationship as well. Molly is quite intelligent herself, but she understands without any resentment that Sherlock's mental prowess is on another level. As a means of levelling the playing field between them, particularly as the series progresses, Molly offsets Sherlock's *intellectual* superiority with her own attempts to assert *moral* superiority. When Sherlock hurts or ignores her, consciously or unconsciously, she immediately corrects him, sometimes with a stern verbal rebuke, such as when he embarrasses her with his deductions in "A Scandal in Belgravia" (S2E1), and goes so far as to slap him across the face when she believes he's taking drugs in "His Last Vow" (S3E3). For his part, Sherlock usually accepts her recriminations, rarely attempting to defend himself, and apologizing with words or a peck on the cheek, or simply letting it pass without comment, especially when his seemingly unfeeling actions are part of a broader gambit to catch a criminal, such as his attempts to confuse his enemies through his real or faked drug use. There's much more trust between Molly and Sherlock than there is with Sherlock and Irene, especially as evidenced through the reliance he places on her discretion in "The Reichenbach Fall" (S2E3), but throughout the series, their relationship is constantly strained by Sherlock's frequent inability to understand how his actions affect Molly, and Molly's inability to openly express her emotions verbally through anything except criticism.

Sherlock has one fake romantic relationship, with Janine (Yasmine Akram), whom he met at John and Mary's wedding. As part of his attempt to bring down the blackmailer Charles Augustus Magnussen, Sherlock begins dating Janine, who works for Magnussen (though she is unaware of his criminal acts), in order to gain access to Magnussen's offices. He even goes so far as to imply that he wants to marry Janine, a step which is taken from the original Conan Doyle story on which "His Last Vow" (S3E3) is loosely based. John's mind is blown when he sees Janine at Sherlock's apartment, having presumably spent the night there, and when John sees the pair kiss, the good doctor gives the impression that he thinks he may be dreaming. Once John realizes Sherlock's true motives in starting a relationship with Janine, he's shocked at how little concern Sherlock has for Janine's feelings. As it turns out, once she learns the truth, Janine is hurt but not heartbroken, at least in what she reveals to Sherlock. Janine gets a bit of revenge by leaking false stories about her kinky love life with Sherlock to the tabloid press, netting a substantial profit from her gossip. In private, it's confirmed that the two have never actually had sex, and Sherlock appears to bear no grudge against Janine for her moneymaking tactic. Janine even says that they might have been friends if Sherlock had handled the situation differently.

Some segments of the fandom have argued that the relationship between Sherlock and Jim Moriarty is actually a romance (a perspective that was winked at with a joking reference in "The Empty Hearse" (S3E1), but more prominent is the innuendo and speculation regarding the relationship between Sherlock and John. From Mrs. Hudson's (Una Stubbs) false assumptions, the possibility of the pair being a couple is the series' longest-running gag, and John's declaration that "I am NOT gay!" is practically his catchphrase. Fanfictions notwithstanding, the relationship between Sherlock and John will be explored more carefully in the upcoming chapter on friendship.

Comparably, both of the Japanese adaptations of Sherlock Holmes portray the detective as completely married to his work. In *Miss Sherlock*, the feminized sleuth never shows any interest in dating or sex whatsoever. In *IQ 246*, the central character is repeatedly urged by his loyal family retainer to marry and produce an heir, but the detective never has any interest in anybody but his female criminal nemesis Maria T (an obvious pun on the original villain), whom he also despises and seeks to defeat. In both cases, the Japanese takes on Holmes put sleuthing first and romance is so far down the list as to be irrelevant.

Jonny Lee Miller's portrayal of Sherlock Holmes on *Elementary* is less clearly – if at all – on the autism spectrum than Downey's, Cumberbatch's, and Takeuchi's. As a diagnosis for Miller's version is much more debatable, he has been left out of this analysis. Unlike almost every other portrayal of Holmes in recent memory, Miller's Holmes is sexually active, with multiple casual partners but hardly any serious romantic relationships over the course of seven seasons. One of his girlfriends, however, is certainly pertinent to this study. Midway through the series, Miller's Holmes develops an interest in Fiona Helbron (Betty Gilpin), a computer programmer with autism. Arguably Fiona's most attractive qualities to Holmes are her frankness and honesty, especially because his most intense previous romantic relationship (with a woman who was a combination of both Irene Adler and Moriarty) was marred by lies. In "Murder Ex Machina" (S4E9), Fiona describes her condition by saying, "They say autism is a spectrum, but it's really an array of different conditions all lumped together." Miller's Holmes begins an awkward courtship with Fiona midway through the series, but she breaks off the relationship after a short while because she gets the feeling that Holmes is treating her less as a girlfriend and more as a project. This leads to a frank and honest conversation in "Ready or Not" (S4E18) where Miller's Holmes discusses his personal insecurities and relationship problems, which wins over Fiona and leads her to initiate a sexual encounter. The relationship continues off-screen for several episodes, but Miller's Holmes breaks it off when he realizes that he will never feel as intensely towards Fiona as he did towards Irene Adler/Jaime Moriarty (Natalie Dormer).

Going beyond Sherlock Holmes, many of the potentially autistic male sleuths are painted as being either uninterested in dating or so socially awkward as to make a lasting relationship challenging, and perhaps improbable. *Law & Order: Criminal Intent's* Robert Goren references having girlfriends and dating in the past, but he never has a serious romantic relationship over the course of the series' run. In the final episode, "To the Boy in the Blue Knit Cap" (S10E8), there's a hint that Goren might consider a relationship with his partner Eames, but Eames' later appearance on an episode of *Law & Order: Special Victims Unit* ("Acceptable Loss," (S14E4)) indicates that nothing came of this. The only woman who expresses having potentially romantic feelings for him is Nicole Wallace (Olivia d'Abo), Goren's nemesis, a manipulator and killer who twists her lovers to achieve her goals. Goren comes up against her several times over the course of the series, but she inevitably escapes official forms of justice – the only time Goren's able to bring her to trial, her wealthy husband funds a defense that gets her acquitted. When Nicole finally meets her demise in "Frame" (S7E22), Goren is informed that her last words were "Tell Bobby he was the only man I ever loved." It's unclear whether Nicole meant these words, or if she was simply trying to get into Goren's head one last time. In any event, Goren never professes to have romantic feelings for her, instead despising her as a sociopathic criminal.

Comparably, Adrian Monk on *Monk* is a widower who is completely devoted to the memory of his late wife. At the heart of *Monk* is the main character's love and loss of his wife, Trudy (Melora Hardin). Before the events of the series, Trudy was killed by a car bomb, causing Monk to have a breakdown and lose his job on the police force. Throughout the series, Monk mourns Trudy, reminisces about their happiest times, and attempts to solve her murder between his other cases. Notably, on the rare occasions when he get angry, it is often when someone speaks disrespectfully of her memory, like in "Mr. Monk is on the Air," (S5E13), when a radio shock jock mocks her brutal death.

On rare occasions, Monk dates again, developing attractions based on characteristics such as how neat and orderly women are. For example, "Mr. Monk and the Other Woman," (S1E7), a woman who maintains the world's cleanest and best-organized garage catches Monk's attention. Monk's attempts at dating never last beyond a single episode and maybe a quick kiss, partly because of his struggles with OCD, mostly because no one can compare to his beloved Trudy.

On *Criminal Minds*, Spencer Reid's social awkwardness is infamous, and few details about his romantic history are known, though it is referenced on occasion that he has a lot of trouble with dating. Despite his frequent efforts, Reid struggles with finding a girlfriend. Reid's longest and most prominent relationship is with geneticist Maeve Donovan (Beth Riesgraf). Their relationship was largely a long-distance one, with most of their interactions taking place over the phone, as Maeve is hiding from a crazed stalker. Unfortunately, the stalker eventually finds and murders Maeve, leaving Reid devastated ("Zugzwang," (S8E12)).

Moving on to *Death Note*, L is not known to have any romantic attachments. In the anime, based on his reaction to a peck on the cheek from Misa, he is attracted to women, though it is unlikely that he could really fall for someone he suspected of being a multiple murderer. Additionally, some fans have some unconfirmed, opinions about the true nature of the feelings between L and Light Yagami, at least on Light's side, based on a few scenes and what Light's name is when spelled backwards. As for all of the live-action adaptations and the musical, no time is devoted to the possibility of L having romantic inclinations. L's near-sole focus, other than snacking on sweets, appears to be his investigations.

In nearly every case save for *Miss Sherlock* and possibly *Detective Sweet*[*], autistic women are all shown in relationships at some point. (Grace Makutsi is not given a boyfriend in the television series *The No. 1 Ladies' Detective Agency*, but she

---

[*] Once again, the lack of English-language subtitles means that *Detective Sweet* cannot be properly analyzed and is included solely for the sake of thoroughness.

does find love and marry in the book series.) Again, in *Miss Sherlock*, Sherlock shows absolutely no signs of interest in romance, or even any attraction to anybody. In the fifth episode, "The Missing Bride," she pours cold water on Wato's musings about perfect weddings, sniping about the number of marriages that end in homicide.

In the filmed play *The Curious Incident of the Dog in the Night-Time*, Christopher shows no interest in having a romantic relationship. He never mentions any desire to find a girlfriend, and the adults in his life do not inquire as to whether he has any interest in dating.

On *King and Maxwell*, Edgar never has a serious relationship on the show, nor is there any mention that he ever dated in the past. There are a few brief scenes that indicate he has an attraction to Benny (Dichen Lachman), a reformed counterfeiter who treats him warmly, but it does not seem that her feelings towards him are romantic. In multiple episodes, Benny spends time with Edgar. Some of her actions might be considered flirtatious, such as when she asks him to bring her a loofah while she's in the shower, and as the scene is played, it seems more like she doesn't view him as a sexual being. When she invites him to lunch at the diner, he considers it a date. Based on the fact that Benny vents to him about her relationship troubles, it seems that she views him strictly as a friend.

Sean Stone on *Chasing Shadows* never shows any signs of attraction to anybody, nor does he voice any interest in a relationship. Indeed, in a misguided attempt to relieve the tension between him and Ruth Hattersley, he bluntly tells her that he doesn't find her attractive, thinking that this will allow them to focus on their work. Not surprisingly, Ruth takes umbrage to the remark.

In the case of Bart Bromley in *The Night Clerk*, what appears to be his first foray into the world of romantic relationships turns out to be a crushing experience. While he's working his hotel job, he meets Andrea Rivera, who treats him with friendliness and obvious respect. Unsurprisingly, Bart is smitten, and after a poolside kiss, he believes that he may have a chance at love, though he's devastated when he realizes that Andrea is in a relationship with a murderer. Bart is willing to change himself to make himself more attractive to Andrea, getting a new haircut, updating his wardrobe, and upgrading his car. When Bart shows Andrea videographic proof that her lover is a killer, she freaks out, and Bart initially thinks he has won her over, but after a seemingly chaste night with her, he soon learns that she has decided to stand by her murdering man, and she has violated his trust by trying to steal the evidence. Though the viewer is not shown all of Bart's emotions, he is never shown to be crushed by Andrea choosing to be an accessory, and turns over additional proofs of guilt to the authorities, leading to the presumed arrest of Andrea and her lover. Andrea seems only mildly disappointed in Bart rather than sharply upset, and her reaction indicates that she's not indignant that Bart was not so infatuated with her that he would let her go. As for Bart, there are no tears or angry outbursts, just a final, brief scene indicating that plans to continue to try to mirror neurotypical behaviors in an attempt to better blend in with the rest of society.

The title character of *Professor T* is fully aware of his awkwardness with dating, though he does wish to change the situation. Over the course of the first few episodes, it is revealed that years earlier, the Professor had a relationship with Christina Brand (Juliet Aubrey), the supervisory officer for the cases he investigates. Though the details are sparse, it's clear that Jasper was very much in love with Christina, but the two broke up, and it's implied that he either deliberately ended the relationship or provoked a breakup because he believed that his mental state would eventually make Christina unhappy. After Christina splits from her husband, the Professor turns to his secretary for dating advice and even goes on a practice date with her before an excruciatingly uncomfortable dinner with Christina, who wishes to pursue a relationship with a different man. As of this writing, the third season of the series has yet to be released, so it remains to be seen what directions the relationship may or may not take.

After all of these examples of romantically awkward or uninterested men, there are very few examples of male sleuths who are potentially on the spectrum who are in lasting, stable relationships. On *CSI*, Gil Grissom begins a relationship with his co-worker Sara Sidle (Jorja Fox), though it's unclear exactly when it began, but it is confirmed in the final scene of the sixth season. The relationship ends when Sara temporarily leaves Las Vegas, but after Gil follows suit at the end of season nine, they marry, but they maintain a long-distance marriage when Sara returns to Las Vegas in season ten. By season thirteen, the pair have separated, with a divorce planned, but they reconcile at the end of the post-series movie "Immortality," and by the time of the spin-off series *CSI: Vegas*, the pair's relationship appears to be strong again.

Doc Martin is one of the rare examples of a character possibly on the spectrum having a successful marriage. For the first half of the series, he has "will-they-won't they" relationship with the local schoolteacher Louisa, eventually getting engaged, breaking off the wedding at the last moment, discovering that Louisa's pregnant, having a son, finally marrying, separating, struggling, reconciling, and then having a daughter. It's not until the last series that their relationship becomes reasonably stable and happy, and the threat of splitting up passes..

Will Graham is about the only character on the spectrum to have a one-night stand, a marriage that arguably ends unhappily, and another complex relationship. In the first season, Will is interested in pursuing a relationship with his colleague Alana Bloom (Caroline Dhavernas), but she rejects him due to what she considers to be his personal hang-ups. The second season features a one-night stand with Margot Verger (Katharine Isabelle), a lesbian who initiated their encounter for the sole purpose of getting pregnant so her child could inherit the family fortune. In the second half of the third season, Will is happily married to Molly (Nina Arianda) and raising her son as his own, but the strain of resuming his work as a criminal profiler strains their relationship. Throughout the series, there's nebulous, unspoken subtext that Will's feelings for Hannibal may have latent romantic undertones.

A couple of characters' approaches to relationships and sexuality change dramatically over time. Sometimes this is portrayed as a natural progression resulting from life experiences, and sometimes these alterations appear to be retcons and sharply deliberate directions of the characters. In the first season of *Dexter*, the title character is completely uninterested in sex and romance. He states that he has had physical relationships in the past, but he doesn't take pleasure in them, and the women's he's been with have always known that there's been something "missing' in his psyche. He pursued a relationship with Rita Bennett (Julie Benz), a woman estranged from her abusive, imprisoned husband, because the trauma from her spouse's cruelty left her uninterested in sex and grateful for the steady, quiet companionship that Dexter could provide. Initially, Dexter seems to be using Rita to create a semblance of normality in his life, though he occasionally seems at a loss at how to act as a boyfriend, and at one point turns to his co-worker Angel Batista (David Zayas) for help, though he soon realizes that he's not looking for assistance in the right direction. Over the course of the first and second seasons, Rita recovers and grows stronger, wanting more from her relationship with Dexter, and the physical aspect of their relationship begins. Both Dexter and Rita's interests in sex awaken over the course of the first two seasons, and by the end of season two, sex is a regular part of their relationship, leading to a pregnancy at the start of season three. Dexter handles the news clumsily at first, but after some reflection he realizes that he wants Rita and her kids in his life, and he proposes, leading to a wedding at the end of season three. It's at this point that his relationship becomes more than just a cover, and instead becomes an integral, even overwhelming part of his life, interfering with his murderous vigilante activities.

At the start of season four, Dexter and Rita have a new baby and are "living the dream" in the suburbs, but as the season progresses, Dexter's dark secrets and lies disrupt their relationship, leading to some emotional turbulence and therapy sessions. Dexter's obsession with learning how Arthur Mitchell (John Lithgow), a decades-active serial killer nicknamed "Trinity" has gotten away with murder for so long leads to disaster. At the end of season four after Dexter passes up multiple opportunities to either kill Mitchell or turn him over to the authorities, Mitchell murders Rita shortly before Dexter kills him, though at the time of Mitchell's death Dexter is unaware of Rita's fate. Dexter discovers Rita's body in a crushing manner, and he's emotionally devastated by her death, and the shadow of his personal guilt at being unable to save her carries on over the course of season five. Only after it is too late does Dexter realize that he is indeed capable of feeling love, and that he had a real chance at happiness with Rita, but he has to bear responsibility for her death due to the consequences of his being a serial killer.

Dexter has four other major romantic relationships over the course of the original series and *New Blood*, aside from three brief flings with women, at least two of which, in season six, may be purely imaginary. The third, at the start of season eight, is only a couple of seconds in a montage. His fling with the unstable artist Lila Tournay (Jaime Murray) is a passionate affair, perhaps the first lust-driven relationship of Dexter's life. It falls apart once Lila's obsession with him turns toxic, and after Lila commits a string of crimes including framing an innocent man for rape, kidnapping, and murder, Dexter inflicts his own dark brand of justice on her, and reunites with Rita afterwards. After Rita's death, Dexter begins a relationship with Lumen Pierce (Julia Stiles) in season five. Lumen is the victim of a gang that preys upon young women, and the season-long storyline where Dexter helps Lumen track down and kill the men who brutalized her is painted as a healing journey for both of them, leading to a romance between them. However, once the last of her tormentors has been slain, Lumen loses interest in killing, and leaves Dexter, as they both realize that she is no longer comfortable in his dark world. In season seven, Hannah McKay (Yvonne Strahovski), a spree killer turned multiple poisoner, is initially the target of one of Dexter's executions, but smitten with mutual lust, the two of them begin an affair, which is briefly ended when Dexter turns Hannah in for trying to kill his sister Debra, but they resume their relationship in season eight. In *New Blood*, Chief of Police Angela Bishop (Julia Jones), has a passionate dating relationship with Dexter, which unravels after she discovers his true identity and proclivities.

In *Murdoch Mysteries*, the love life of Llwellyn Watts changes dramatically over the course of the series. Watts has no serious romantic relationships over his first appearances seasons ten through twelve, but that all changes dramatically when he his character is abruptly revealed to be gay in the thirteenth season. Based on an interview with the showrunners on the season thirteen DVD, they decided to make Watts gay after he'd already been on the show for a few seasons, with the enthusiastic support of Daniel Maslany. This characterization is confounded a bit by the fact that in earlier seasons, Watts is shown to be attracted to women, chiefly the bicyclist Fiona Faust (Kelly McNamee) in "Brackenreid Boudoir" (S11E8), whom he kisses before she continues on her journey. In other episodes, such as "The Accident," (S11E7), Watts is shown being awkward around attractive women, looking (though not leering) at them in a discomfited manner. In these early episode, he's the stereotypical romantically clumsy Aspie type, clearly more comfortable in the world of intellectual ideas than with other people.

It's not until "The Philately Fatality" that Watts begins a relationship with a man, taking the initiative in reaching out to Jack Walker (Jesse Lavercombe), a butcher who's trying to hide his sexuality. Their relationship lasts on and off for the next few seasons, interrupted by Walker marrying a pregnant woman as a cover, during which time Watts befriends the bon vivant Milo Strange (David Andrew Reid). After the murder of Walker's wife by her ex-lover, Walker flees to New York to begin a new life, temporarily followed by Watts, but after a brief period of domesticity, Watts decides his path lies elsewhere. After his return to Toronto, he has at least one relationship with an anonymous unseen man, and becomes an outspoken proponent for gay rights, to the extent that it is possible at that time.

The main issue with Watts' relationship development is the abruptness of it. Had more foreshadowing been present, the transition from romantic awkwardness to more confident dating in a society that largely disapproves of same-sex relationships would not be so jarring. There's no segue, and his previous attractions to women are forgotten, as an attempt at conversion therapy suggests that he can't feel any attraction to women at all.

Murdoch Mysteries' retconning of the love lives of its potentially autistic detectives carries over to the title character as well. Murdoch's love life is initially devoid of physical aspects, as he is a deeply religious practicing Catholic. He was engaged prior to the events of the series, but his fiancée passed away. Throughout the series, his primary love interest is Julia Ogden (Hélène Joy), a doctor whose opinions on most issues differ strongly from his own, but he's strongly attracted to her intelligence and their shared interests. Drama follows over the next several seasons, as they date on and off, Julia marries someone else, followed by separation, the murder of her husband, her conviction and near-execution for the crime before Murdoch saves her, and their eventual marriage in the hundredth episode, followed by a baby girl several seasons later. It's a happy, strong, stable marriage, interrupted briefly by severe arguments over Julia's involvement in abortion and euthanasia, issues that Murdoch says they'll need to talk through, but these discussions are never shown on-screen.

During his "off" periods with Julia in the early seasons, Murdoch briefly sees a widow with a son, and he meets a woman, Anna Fulford (Lisa Faulkner) with whom he is compatible, but she realizes that his true love lies elsewhere. At the time they meet ("The Murdoch Identity," (S3E1)), Murdoch has amnesia. For a decade, it's portrayed as a completely innocent relationship, but at the end of season fourteen, the showrunners apparently wanted to introduce a son for Murdoch, and they retconned "The Murdoch Identity" to suggest that the amnesia made him forget his sexual morality as well, leading to a child that for whatever reason, Anna never mentioned to him during their occasional meetings over the next few years. It's a clumsy way to provide Murdoch with the son he always wanted, at an age where the boy is old enough to be involved in the storylines.

As for the women on the spectrum, several of them are shown to be very casual towards sex, though the ones that marry tend to have stable relationships. Just like the men, there is a diverse mix of relationship statuses, though there is one crucial recurring difference. Men on the autism spectrum are often (not always) told that they need to change, usually by acting in a more neurotypical manner, if they want to find a mate, like in *The Night Clerk*, where Bart gives himself a makeover and self-taught lessons in social interaction in order to pursue his romantic interest. William Murdoch has to suppress or compromise his personal convictions on multiple occasions if he wants to stay married to Julia Ogden. Martin Ellingham has to radically revise the way he expresses affection and communicates to save his marriage, Dexter Morgan has to hide his Dark Passenger (of course, this change is needed for very different reasons), and Will Graham concludes that he has to shut himself off from his preternatural criminal profiling powers if he's ever going to enjoy a happy marriage to Molly. Some of the personal traits that define them as individuals must be suppressed or altered if they want a lasting relationship.

Autistic women, in contrast, attract partners who like them in spite of or perhaps because they are different, and while they may need to adjust their understanding of what their partner needs and wants, they never feel compelled to change their mannerisms, personal styles, or anything distinctive about their characters in order to be more desirable. Their mates have to accept them as they are.

On *24*, Chloe O'Brian has four known romantic relationships. She has a one-night stand at the start of the fourth season, which she seems to regret, and she has no significant feelings for the man. At some point prior to the start of season six, she recently ended a brief relationship with a co-worker, who wants to continue the relationship, but she's firm in asserting that's she finished with dating him, though she wishes to maintain a cordial and professional working relationship. Her major relationship over the series is with Morris O'Brian (Carlo Rota). He's introduced at the end of season five as Chloe's ex-husband, and while he's warm to her, she's best described as "not hostile," and they work well together, even going out to breakfast at the end of the season. At some point before season six and at some point before or after Chloe dating another co-worker, they had sex, and she revealed her pregnancy at the end of season six. They remarry and have a son and an apparently happy relationship for seasons seven and eight. Unfortunately, Morris and their son, Prescott, are presumably killed in a car crash after the events of season eight (though on *24*, death is not always a permanent condition), and Chloe becomes convinced that they were assassinated by retaliatory government agents. This leads her to begin dating Adrian Cross (Michael Wincott), a freedom of information activist who revels in hacking and revealing government secrets in *24: Live Another Day*. As it turns out, Cross determined that Morris's and Prescott's deaths were most likely accidents, but he withheld this information from Chloe, presumably to keep her angry towards the U.S. government and loyal to him and his cause. This manipulation is never addressed at length, as Cross is killed by a terrorist moments later.

Chloe's relationship with Morris is far and away her most important and stable romantic pairing on the series. It's notable that Morris doesn't ask her to adjust anything major about herself, though Chloe does insist that Morris address his most serious issue: his alcoholism. A significant subplot in season six revolves around Morris battling his urge to drink, but this struggle is one that both individuals are concerned with addressing. At one point, Chloe kisses Morris for the sole purpose of testing his breath for alcohol, and he resents the implied lack of trust. Otherwise, their bond appears to be fairly devoid of drama on a personal level.

Temperance Brennan is one of the few characters discussed in this book to have a successful romantic relationship. In the early seasons, she dates occasionally, with the relationship often becoming sexual. Midway through the series, the friendly albeit sometimes turbulent working relationship with Seeley Booth grows romantic, the two consummate their relationship at the end of season six, which leads to a daughter born the following season, and their marriage in season eight, with a son being born between the interval of the tenth and eleventh seasons.

Lisbeth Salander has both male and female sex partners, but the depth of her emotional ties to them is kept vague in the films. It's suggested that at the end of the English-language version of *The Girl with the Dragon Tattoo* that Lisbeth was interested in pursuing a more serious relationship with Mikael Blomkvist (Daniel Craig), even buying him an expensive custom-made leather jacket for Christmas, but she trashes the present before giving it to him when she realizes that he is still in a relationship with his editor. Otherwise, her romantic relationships in the movies are mostly with women, and though her girlfriends all seem fond of her, the level of emotional intimacy on Lisbeth's part is portrayed minimally on-screen. The depth and intensity of Lisbeth's feelings for anybody is mainly viewer conjecture. With all three actresses playing the role, Lisbeth's personal emotions depend on how people read her facial expressions in various situations. Because of this, there's a touch of irony in the fact that people with certain forms of autism have more difficulty interpreting Lisbeth's feelings.

In the original *The Bridge*, Saga is open about how much she enjoys sex, and early in the series, when she finds herself desiring a tryst, she goes to a crowded bar and catches the eye of a man. When he asks her if he can buy her a drink, she declines, and feeling rejected, he walks away. Confused, she follows him, explaining that she wasn't interested in a drink, but she wants him to go back to her place for sex. The man is stunned, but he follows her home. They have sex again later, and she seems content for their relationship to be based entirely on casual hook-ups, but he's interested in actually building an emotional connection to her, and suggests dates to get to know each other better. The initial pick-up scene and relationship arc are replicated pretty faithfully in the American version.

The relationship doesn't last long, as by the second season of the Scandinavian *The Bridge*, Saga has moved in with a different boyfriend. However, she soon learns that she doesn't like his intrusions on her privacy, and she throws out his things (he's later able to retrieve them), not realizing how this annoys him, and she checks into a hotel for a night so as to have alone time. Later in the season, her boyfriend realizes that she can't provide the kind of relationship he wants, and he leaves. In series three, Saga begins a relationship with her new Danish partner, Henrik Sabroe (Thure Lindhardt), and it continues throughout the fourth season, with the possibility of it developing further left open, thanks to how she helped him heal from his emotional traumas after reuniting him with his long-lost daughter.

As for Sonya in the American version, she has one other relationship with a man over a few episodes of the second season – Jack Dobbs (Nathan Phillips) – the brother of the man who killed her sister, of all people. They meet at the prison hospital, where Sonya's sister's killer is dying, and it leads to a casual hook-up, which then continues despite her superior officer and father figure Lieutenant Hank Wade's (Ted Levine) insistence that no good can come from it. Eventually, Jack reveals that he knew his brother had killed another woman before Sonya's sister, and Sonya ends the relationship because she knows she cannot trust him.

Once again, the production team of *The Tunnel* has indicated that they were trying to refocus their female lead's mannerisms outside of an autistic interpretation, but there are still several autistic indicators in Posey's portrayal. At the same time, some of the classic moments featuring Saga's bluntness and inability to understand nuance are heavily toned down or removed. *The Tunnel* alters the infamous bar pick-up scene in season one, changing it into a quieter conversation without the confusion arising from the female lead's directness and failure to understand how her refusal of a drink could be misinterpreted. In the second series, Elise is dating a man named Gaël (Thibaul Evrard), who supports her personal idiosyncrasies, but her constant prioritizing her investigating over time with him leads to a breakup, and she begins a lesbian relationship with Eryka (Laura de Boer), a suspect in the central case. The showrunners give the pair comparable tragedies in their backstories as a means of creating a bond, but once it's revealed that Eryka is indeed partially responsible for many deaths, *The Tunnel's* showrunners take the plotline into a direction that damages the moral compass of Elise and the show as a whole. When Eryka proudly declares that she took the side she deemed "less hypocritical," Elise never calls her out for the murders, and even Karl, who was so upset about the deaths of innocent children a few episodes earlier, has forgotten his moral outrage. The series' attempts to justify terrorist actions, as they did in the previous season, damages the moral tone of the show, as it consciously or unconsciously teaches the horrible lesson that violent terrorism is an acceptable means of social change. Rather than having Elise recoil in horror at having fallen for a psychopath and rejecting Eryka, the relationship ends by Eryka running away, and the closing scenes show Elise having a romantic dream about her and Eryka. In series three, Elise's bisexuality is reinforced with a quick mention that she had her first sexual experience with a boy at the age of thirteen, and her first affair with a girl came two years later.

    Holly Gibney is shown taken the initiative in starting a relationship in the second season of *Mr. Mercedes*, where Lupe's Holly strongly suggests to an autistic man she knows from a therapy group that she'd be interested a date with him. No scenes of them as a couple are shown, and clearly the relationship doesn't work out, as in the third season Roland Finkelstein (Brett Gelman), a defense attorney, develops feelings for Holly, and they are shown dating at the end of the season, though hardly any details are given about their relationship. In *The Outsider*, Erivo's Holly meets police officer turned security specialist Andy Katcavage (Derek Cecil), and he seems smitten with her soon after they first meet. He asks her out, though notably he seems more nervous and awkward than she is, and they go out a few times. At one point, he stays in her hotel room, but nothing clear is shown as to whether their relationship turns physical or not. When Katcavage is killed at the season's end, Erivo's Holly is clearly badly shaken and hurt by his death.

In *Astrid et Raphaëlle,* Astrid recognizes that her autism has impaired her ability to begin a relationship, and her friendship with Raphaëlle and her support group are critical in her learning new behaviors and guidance in pursuing relationships. Astrid is the driving force in her own attempts at self-improvement. By season two, she has begun dating Tetsuo Tanaka (Kengo Saito), but their relationship is often tailored to fit Astrid's own personal comfort zone. In "Le Livre" (S2E7), Astrid and Tetsuo spend time together, which appears to consist almost entirely on sitting on a park bench in silence. From the smile on Astrid's face, she's completely happy with what they're doing.

Finally, one of the leading subplots of the first season of *Extraordinary Attorney Woo* centers around Woo Young-Woo's relationship with Lee Jun-ho (Kang Tae-oh), a private investigator working for Hanbada. Lee Jun-ho is arguably the most eligible bachelor at Hanbada, and he's the constant target of attention and flirtation by the young women who also work there. Having his choice of girlfriends, Lee Jun-ho finds himself drawn to Woo Young-Woo, whom he meets when she's having trouble walking through the revolving door of the office building. He kindly provides advice rather than mockery, and as they work together, he becomes impressed by her legal knowledge and personality. While others are annoyed by Woo Young-Woo's constant talking about whales, Lee Jun-ho enjoys it… in moderation. As they begin dating, Lee Jun-ho provides gentle, supportive advice as she navigates the previously unknown territory, such as kissing (their physical content never goes beyond brief kissing and handholding in the first season), and when she becomes obsessed with her personal fascinations, he's mostly patient as he suggests adjustments to their dates to reshape them into activities that they both can enjoy, instead of centering solely around Woo Young-Woo's mainly whale-based interests. Woo Young-Woo breaks off the relationship after overhearing Lee Jun-ho's sister's comments that he'd be stuck caring for someone with a disability. The remark cuts Woo Young-Woo deeply, and she believes that staying in the relationship will lead to Lee Jun-ho eventually resenting her. After Lee Jun-ho makes it clear that his sister doesn't speak for him, and Woo Young-Woo realizes that she can be in a relationship without becoming a burden to her partner, they reconcile in the season one finale.

Notably, all of the characters in these productions are portrayed as being fully willing and active partners in any romantic relationships they may have. There are no cases of a naïve_person with autism being exploited or manipulated in a relationship, a possibility that many parents worry about in real life. Woo Young-Woo's father is concerned about his daughter's dating, but in the case of the extremely caring and respectful Lee Jun-ho his worries are unfounded.

There's no denying that romance can be challenging for neurotypical people as well, and characters in dramatic productions are often given more opportunities to find love and more understanding and accepting partners than people with autism do in real life. In the second season of *Big Little Lies*, the character Jane Chapman (Shailene Woodley), tells Bonnie Carlson (Zoë Kravitz), that her new boyfriend has some light autistic qualities, to which Bonnie replies that she's heard that some guys fake being autistic as a means of picking up women. No further details are given, but surely some real-life autistic men watched that scene and thought, "Really? Are there women who are attracted to men with autism? And if so, can you please introduce me to them?" Few of these series, with the possible exception of *Criminal Minds*, really delve into how when autism can impair one's ability to form romantic relationships, the emotional effect on the autistic person can be devastating.

CHAPTER NINE
But You've Got to Have Friends

Romantic relationships can be intensely difficult for people on the spectrum. Friendships often bring challenges of their own, and though friendship is usually less fraught with drama than romance, it can still be daunting for many people on the spectrum. It can be arduous to build connections with other people when social situations are overwhelming, or when solitude is the most familiar and comfortable state for an autistic person.

Looking at the characters discussed in this study, none of them can be considered popular socially. Very few of them are shown having friends outside of work, and with very few exceptions, the autistic sleuths' social circles tend to revolve entirely around their investigative teams. Most of their friends are co-workers... when they have friends at all.

A handful of the characters analyzed here barely have any amicable connections with anyone at all outside their immediate families, though they are rarely shown complaining or wishing they were more popular. The emotions behind their facial expressions, however, are often open to debate. Christopher Boone in *The Curious Incident of the Dog in the Night-Time* has no friends his age, and aside from his relationships with parents and teachers, his closest companion is his pet rat. He cannot connect emotionally with any of his classmates, as his school is filled with students with a wide assortment of developmental disabilities that are in some ways more severe than his own. Christopher lives in a no-man's land, denied the chance to meet people his own age with comparable intelligence, and surrounded by atypical youths with whom he cannot build intellectual or emotional connections. In the filmed play, Christopher is not shown confiding in anybody directly, but all of his personal thoughts are written into a diary which is then read by his teacher. Christopher's only outlet for an emotional release is through the written word.

Along similar lines, Sean Stone in *Chasing Shadows* lives a nearly solitary life outside of work, and though his housekeeper cares for him like an older sister, they do not share a traditional friendship, and Sean's relationships with all of his co-workers are too tense to be considered friendships. Perhaps he might have developed closer connections with his co-workers in time, but the show's cancellation after the four-episode first series means that that the character will never be shown forming real friendships. The title character in *Professor T* has colleagues in the police force and the university, but none of them qualify as pals, and he never relaxes with anybody for purely social reasons. Bart Bromley in *The Night Clerk* is similarly friendless, having no supportive presence in his life other than his mother. Lisbeth Salander works alongside Mikael Blomkvist and has a brief fling with him, but is she really friends with Mikael or any of her female sexual partners? On various occasions she appears to show affection or concern for them, but there are no scenes with them outside of investigative work or having non-carnal fun, nor does she discuss her personal issues with them. As Lisbeth expresses her emotions differently from most people, it's possible that she considers them friends, and certainly they care about her, but based solely on what's portrayed on-screen, the viewer doesn't see much evidence of genuine reciprocal friendship.

It should be stressed that there are varying levels of friendships. Everybody, neurotypical on the spectrum, or anywhere else, may consider that they have a small number of very close friends, a larger circle of friendly acquaintances, a certain number of people they socialize with because they have to and not because they like them, individuals with whom they maintain an amicable relationship with at their jobs and never see outside the workplace, and any number of other categorizations. And neurotypical people can enjoy time on their own just as much as the autistic. However, there is a general trend in the entertainment industry discussed here that places the autistic in solitary positions more often, with limited camaraderie.

In some cases, the extent of the isolation in the sleuths' lives is debatable. Martin Ellingham in *Doc Martin* is surrounded by villagers who consider him a friend, though it often seems that he doesn't reciprocate their feelings, though by the final episode, it's clear that he has developed a deep affection for Portwenn, and that includes the people in it. Though all of supporting cast grow to like and care about him, Martin does not socialize for pleasure or share feelings with any of them. As much as he loves his wife, Louisa, it's challenging for him to express his emotions to her. His only real confidants are his aunts, particularly the trained mental health professional, Aunt Ruth, in the later series. L in *Death Note* famously declares that Light Yagami may be his very first friend, though there's a strong implication that this statement is a lie meant to manipulate Light. All of L's conversations and shared investigative interactions with Light are tainted by the fact true friendship depends on trust, and L always suspects that Light is a serial killer. It is possible that the two could have been genuine friends, as evidenced by the period where Light's mind has been magically erased of the memory of his crimes, but at all other times Light views L as an opponent to be vanquished., further precluding real friendship. L does have a close relationship with his guardian turned assistant Watari (in every version of *Death Note* except the musical, where Watari has been deleted), but the connection may not be one of equal friendship so much as is it a blend of a guardian/ward relationship and an employer/assistant relationship. Only in the live-action miniseries does Yamazaki's L have a genuine emotional connection with one character – Near (Mio Yûki) – who is portrayed more of a little sibling than a friend.

Notably, none of these characters shows any disappointment whatsoever at lacking close friends. There are no tears or whines about being unpopular, nor do any of them seek counsel on how to change their social status, nor do they try to find a pal or enter an existing social group. Their absence of connections is simply accepted and treated stoically, and it's debatable as to whether any of them considers friendlessness to be a problem at all. Of course, the necessities of keeping the plot moving and other dramatic concerns mean that certain aspects of characterization may be minimized – after all, the power of a high-speed chase after a multiple murderer in *Death Note* would be diluted if L stopped flying the helicopter so he could whine about his feelings.

Looking at the vast majority of the sleuths on the spectrum, the overwhelming number of their friends solve crimes alongside them. In all of the police procedural shown here, the autistic sleuths' social lives seem to revolve entirely around their jobs. Virtually everyone they trust is a member of the investigative team. Of course, part of this is a conceit of television shows, where characters' lives center around the central cast, but it is still a trend affecting how the general public views the autistic. Like everybody else, autistic people may find comfort in keeping company with people who hold similar values, such as strong senses of justice.

A recurring trope amongst the autistic sleuths is how stunned– and not necessarily delighted– they are to discover that they have made one genuine friend. This revelation often is presented as a climactic emotional moment, though the audience is well-aware that the connection between the two characters has become a friendship long before the autistic character has come to that realization.

The Holmes-Watson pairing is far and away one of the most famous friendships in all of literature, and it's at the heart of both the Downey and Cumberbatch Holmes series. Watson is Holmes' chronicler and assistant, and is essential to Holmes' success as a detective. Both the Law and the Freeman Watsons are often exasperated by Holmes' atypical behavior, but the friendships continue due to the bonds between the men, built not just out of caring for each other as people, but for the thrill of the chase that comes with investigation. There are big emotional moments where the importance of the Watson/Holmes friendship permeates both franchises. Midway through the first Downey *Sherlock Holmes*, Watson is injured in an explosion, and when a disguised on-the-lam Holmes visits his bedridden friend in the hospital, Mary Morstan (Kelly Reilly) sees through the makeup at once, and the brief pause in the action is the most poignant moment of the film, as all attempts at flippancy are shoved aside, and Holmes shows nothing but pure, genuine, devastated concern. Likewise, in *Sherlock's* "The Hounds of Baskerville," (S2E2), the key emotional moment comes after Sherlock tells Watson that he doesn't have friends. Watson's hurt, but later, Sherlock clarifies it by saying "I don't have friends. I've just got one." The identity of that sole friend is obvious to John, and though he doesn't provide much in the way of reaction, the importance of that remark is not lost on him. The friendship's importance to Sherlock is further emphasized through Sherlock's distress during their brief falling-outs in "The Empty Hearse" (S3E1) and the more serious rift in "The

Lying Detective" (S4E2). *Sherlock's* "The Final Problem" (S4E3) takes Sherlock's personal categorization of his friendship even further, as Sherlock identifies him as family, a remark that John silently but clearly appreciates through his facial expression. The last episode to date of *Sherlock* tries to give an additional potential psychological hang-up explaining Sherlock's difficulty at forming friendships beyond autism, indicating that the trauma from his childhood best pal's disappearance may have warped his social skills.

Throughout *Miss Sherlock*, it almost becomes a recurring gag as to how often Sherlock informs a third party at least once an episode that she and Wato are not friends. In *Miss Sherlock*, Sherlock and Wato are brought together by chance during the investigation of the murder of Wato's former mentor, and Sherlock's brother Kento (Yukiyoshi Ozawa) suggests that Wato, needing a place to stay, room with Sherlock, claiming that he'll feel better with someone looking after his sister. Sherlock isn't pleased with this plan, and is deliberately rude to Wato in the second episode, refusing Wato's elaborate home-cooked breakfast, forcing a long list of rules upon her new roommate, and generally being ornery in the hopes of driving away Wato. Over the next several episodes, she frequently treats Wato as an annoying servant, and rarely misses a chance to contradict Wato or to compare Wato's intelligence negatively to her own. Yet, as the series progresses, the two develop an effective investigative relationship, and by the final episode, when Wato is brainwashed into becoming a killer, Sherlock successfully deprograms her by stating the unspoken obvious in the biggest emotional moment of the show, that Wato is indeed Sherlock's friend, the first she's ever had.

Similarly, on the Scandinavian *The Bridge*, Saga has no real friends outside work. She's very close to her supervisor,

Hans Petterson (Dag Malmberg), who's like a surrogate father to her, but she has no other close relationships with any of her other colleagues on the Swedish police force. The only other co-worker who treats her warmly is the unnamed pathologist (Gabriel Flores Jair), and they have precious little interaction outside the mortuary. Her sole platonic friendship is in the first two seasons, with her Danish investigative partner Martin Rohde (Kim Bodnia), although she gets off to a hostile start with him at the beginning of their investigation, but they grow closer, building trust and respect as they hunt a serial killer. Notably, they have no interaction for over a year between seasons one and two. This is portrayed on-screen as the fault of the socially awkward Saga, but there was nothing preventing Martin from initiating contact besides his own emotional turmoil after his son was murdered at the end of season one. Throughout the first two seasons, both try to help the other with personal issues. Martin provides suggestions on how to work better with people, tips that often strike Saga as illogical and useless. In contrast, Saga provides characteristically blunt observations as to how Martin messes up his own life and wounds his family through his selfishness and angst. Martin is generally offended, though from his facial expressions, he can see the justice in her remarks.

The two become a better team as the second season progresses, but their relationship culminates at the end of season two, when Martin is implied to have poisoned the man who killed his son. Saga figures out what happened, and she's faced with a moral choice. As she tells Martin, he is her only friend. It's clear that the thought of sending him to prison is crushing to Saga, but despite how much she cares for Martin, she informs the police of her suspicions and Martin is arrested and presumably convicted. For Saga, her conscience is more important than her friendship with Martin. Earlier, Martin tried to teach the often offensively honest Saga how to lie in social situations, but ultimately, the truth and personality morality are what is most important to Saga. As much as she cares about Martin, she cannot become an accessory after the fact because he has once again succumbed to his destructive impulses. This exemplifies the adherence to a strict moral code and rigidity that is often seen as a hallmark of the autistic. Viewers may be split on how they view Saga's choice, but the series seems to argue she is more concerned about being a good person than she is about being a supposedly good friend.

    The autistic characters may sometimes have difficulty realizing what constitutes being a good friend to someone else, but their associates often realize what needs to be done in order to be a good friend to their autistic compatriots. In a handful of cases, the closest friends of the autistic sleuths play pivotal roles in helping the detectives navigate society. In these cases, the friends serve as guides to the neurotypical world. Certainly, Watson is the most famous example. Especially on *Sherlock*, Watson often pours oil on the troubled waters when Sherlock has been particularly abrasive, and frequently nudges Sherlock to modify his behavior.

    In one case, *Monk*, Adrian Monk actually has to hire an assistant to help him navigate the more difficult aspects of social life. Sharona Fleming (Bitty Schram) and Natalie Teeger (Traylor Howard) are his paid assistants, ostensibly to help him handle issues connected with his OCD such as handing him hand wipes, but in practice, they also help with all manner of social customs as well that might challenge the autistic. Monk has no prominent friends outside of his investigative circle. This point is emphasized in "Mr. Monk Makes a Friend" (S5E11), where Hal Tucker (Andy Richter), is a murderer who needs to retrieve incriminating information that has been mailed to Monk, so he pretends to befriend Monk until he gets his hands on what he wants, after which point he ghosts him. It's notable that all of the other members of the main cast are suspicious of Hal, and they act as if no one could possibly want to be Monk's friend voluntarily, which is an uncharacteristically insensitive moment for them. The redemptive moment comes after the end, when Monk and the rest of the gang arrest Hal for murder, and Captain Stottlemeyer (Ted Levine) declares that Monk is his friend. The friendship between the two men is one of the backbones of the series. After the first season, where Monk was primarily a source of annoyance for Stottlemeyer, the relationship was rewritten to emphasize no matter how much Monk may drive Stottlemeyer off the wall, he likes Monk and deeply respects his investigative skills and his persistence in trying to survive in the wake of his mental illness. Both men have a strong emotional investment in seeing murderers receive their comeuppance.

    Other cases where the main character's best friend serves as a guide to the neurotypical world include the titular Astrid, where the investigative partnership between Astrid and Raphaëlle is based on Raphaëlle assisting Astrid socially in exchange for access to Astrid's research skills. Frequently, Temperance Brennan's best friend, Angela Montenegro (Michaela Conlin), takes it upon herself to provide tips on everything from popular culture to how best to respond to another person. Comparably, Precious Ramotswe (Jill Scott) serves as Grace Makutsi's mentor, providing her perspective on human nature to guide her along in the investigations. And on *Mr. Mercedes*, Justine Lupe's Holly Gibney receives similar direction on detective work and understanding other people from Bill Hodges (Brendan Gleason). All of these instances show how gentle guidance from a caring friend can provide appreciable benefits to a person on the spectrum, providing useful assistance without being patronizing or hurtful.

The autistic sleuths may get most of their companionship from the people they work with, with scarce exceptions. Of all the characters in this study, only one autistic sleuth has a longtime friend outside of their work/investigative circles, with the proviso that the friend in question is a significant member of the production's cast. Murdoch on *Murdoch Mysteries*, for example, befriends some historical figures like Nikola Tesla (Dmitry Chepovetsky), and has a childhood friend, Freddie Pink (Alex Paxton-Beesley), who grew up to become a private investigator, but these characters appear rarely, and he does not share deep personal feelings with them. His closest friendship is with his subordinate Constable George Crabtree (Jonny Harris), whose enthusiastic embrace of outlandish possibilities and imagination stand in sharp contrast to Murdoch's sober, logical practicality. Despite their differences, the pair have an excellent working relationship and are very close.

Only Woo Young-Woo on *Extraordinary Attorney Woo* has a long-term friend outside of work who is a major character. Dong Geu-ra-mi (Joo Hyun-young), befriended Woo Young-Woo when they were at school together, and their emotional connection grew. In the fourth episode, "The Strife of the Three Brothers," it is revealed that both Woo Young-Woo and Dong Geu-ra-mi were outsiders at their school, with Woo Young-Woo's autism making her the target of bullying, and Dong Geu-ra-mi being a deliberate nonconformist. Dong Geu-ra-mi lashed out at Woo Young-Woo's bullies at one point, and Woo Young-Woo suggested that they become friends, as neither had any other buddies. At first, Dong Geu-ra-mi seemed incredulous at the idea that the two of them could form a bond, but their friendship matured and endured.

At first glance the two have little in common. Woo Young-Woo is quiet, studious, and devoted to her law work. Dong Geu-ra-mi is eccentric, unafraid of drawing attention to herself, and makes her living as a waitress. But the two routinely greet each other with their own ritual, neither ever criticizes the other, and both turn to each other with their problems. Dong Geu-ra-mi is not part of the Hanbada law firm group, and in several episodes she only appears briefly in order to discuss Woo Young-Woo's problems with her, but she plays larger roles when she needs Woo Young-Woo to represent her father in a legal matter, or when she and her boss at the restaurant join the Hanbada team on a business trip as their personal cooks, though her assistance in solving cases is minimal. Dong Geu-ra-mi's friendship is a constant source of support and comfort for Woo Young-Woo, and it shows how an autistic person can maintain a deep and supportive friendship with a very different neurotypical person outside of work. Both appreciate and value the qualities that the other brings to the friendship.

Social awkwardness is widely considered to be a hallmark of autism, but all of these shows take that issue and expand it to levels that make their subjects appear not just isolated, but almost pitiable in their loneliness, at least in the eyes of many neurotypical viewers. Once again, most of these characters are portrayed as being comfortable with the size and intensity of their social circles. In most of these cases, it's suggested that these characters' lives revolve entirely around their employment, and any entertainment pursuits outside of work are strictly solitary endeavors, such as model airplanes, jigsaw puzzles, and reading. Certainly there is a level of realism here for many people with autism– but this level of limited friendship is by no means universal, so what does it mean such depictions are so widespread in dramatizations?

CHAPTER TEN
The Autistic Perpetrator

So far, this book has focused on how autistic minds are portrayed as skilled at crime-solving. But what happens when an autistic person *commits* a crime? Do the mental processes that supposedly help them with detection also make them better criminals? Or do the issues that cause them problems with their everyday lives affect their ability to get away with misdeeds?

As the following examples will illustrate, portrayals of the autistic as criminals are a mixed bag, sometimes relying too heavily on the then-widely accepted misconception that having autism meant that one lacked the ability to feel empathy. The earliest examples were written during a time when understandings of Asperger's Syndrome were just entering the mainstream consciousness, and as such, they lack some of the nuance and complexity of later characterizations. I wish to stress that even though at times the writing and characterization may be a bit lacking in earlier scripts, in most of these cases, the acting itself is quite well done.

This is of course not an extensive list of autistic perpetrators, but I have put special focus on the shows and franchises discussed elsewhere in this book, with a particularly notable example from an additional series, the British legal drama *The Brief*.

Law & Order: CI – Wally Stevens (Mark Linn-Baker) (2003)

In this episode, Goren and Eames investigate the brutal death of a homeless man, and discover that the victim is one of sixteen recently killed homeless people, all of whose lives were insured for massive sums. As the detectives need help understanding the complexities of the insurance industry, insurance man Wally Stevens is recruited to help them study the cases. Initially, Goren takes a liking to Wally, who has pronounced autistic mannerisms and speech patterns. Wally's habits are like magnified versions of Goren's, and after their first meeting with Wally, Eames quips to Goren, "I didn't know you had an older, geekier brother." As the case progresses, Goren realizes that the only person with the know-how to devise a multi-million dollar insurance scam is Wally himself, and Goren goes further, diagnosing Wally with Asperger's Syndrome. Wally's wife recently left him for a much wealthier man. She gained full custody of their two sons, leaving Wally alone and desperate, believing that he needed to obtain a huge sum of money in order to win back his ex-wife. Wally arranged for fifteen people to be killed in the insurance scheme, and he slew one of his partners in crime when his confederate went rogue and murdered an additional, unplanned homeless person.

When the detectives confront Wally in the lonely house where he once lived with his family, they subtly manipulate him into revealing the unconscious patterns he creates, and confront him with the fact that he has lost his family, which he has not been able to admit to anybody else. When Wally is told what Asperger's Syndrome entails, it causes a meltdown, and a visibly distraught Wally screams, declaring that the symptoms fit him perfectly and begs to know why no one ever thought to inform him of his condition. Eames shows much more compassion than she usually does to killers when she explains the newness of the diagnosis, and Goren shows none of the disgust that is standard when he arrests murderers. It's the diagnosis that crumbles all of Wally's defenses, and he makes a full confession.

Wally Stevens stands out amongst the *Criminal Intent* perpetrators as one of the most sympathetically portrayed killers. The reason for this is due almost entirely to his autism, and the negative effects that it/ has. He is responsible for far more deaths than most of the series' other villains. Though he only killed one man directly, his involvement in the insurance scam led to the deaths of fifteen homeless people. Incidentally, given Wally's intelligence and knowledge of the insurance industry, it shouldn't have been hard for him to come up with an alternative plan for insurance fraud that didn't involve multiple murder, such as the supposed theft or destruction of valuable artwork or something similar. There's an important stylistic choice here, as the only two human victims shown on-screen are the one victim of the insurance fraud whose death was completely unconnected to Wally, and Wally's murderous partner in crime, who is the only person Wally killed directly. The fifteen murdered homeless people are never shown onscreen, except for a brief glimpse of a photograph, most aren't named, and none of their characters are developed. By keeping the victims to an abstraction, they seem less real to the viewer and therefore, Wally's crimes have less resonance, minimizing the horrific nature of his deeds for those viewers who don't take the time to think too deeply about the narrative.

Law & Order: SVU & Law & Order: Trial by Jury – Gabriel Duvall (Alfred Molina) (2005)

In a pair of crossover episodes, "Night" (*SVU*, (S6E20)), and "Day," (*Trial by Jury*, (S1E11)), the NYPD detectives investigate a multiple rapist who targets marginalized women. Eventually, the perpetrator is revealed to be Gabriel Duvall, a computer expert and a member of a wealthy and prominent family. In the middle of his trial, Gabriel is diagnosed with Asperger's Syndrome.

To its credit, "Day" makes a point of stressing that Gabriel's serial rapes are not a direct product of his Asperger's

Syndrome. After the clinical psychologist Dr. Elizabeth Olivet (Carolyn McCormick) examines Gabriel, Olivet reports back to the ADA Tracey Kibre (Bebe Neuwirth), that she does believe that Gabriel has Asperger's, and that the reason why he wasn't diagnosed earlier is because Asperger's was widely unknown until very recently. Olivet stresses that being on the autism spectrum did not contribute to Gabriel's condition, and that people with autism are much more likely to be victims of serious crimes than perpetrators. Aside from suggesting that sexual contact between a young Gabriel and a member of the domestic staff may have triggered some of his behaviors, Olivet provides no explanation or diagnosis for the reasons why Gabriel became a serial rapist, nor does she explore the question as to whether he can control his behavior. This leads to a slightly convoluted portrait of Gabriel's psyche. Essentially, Olivet is saying that Gabriel has Asperger's, that the Asperger's is not the root cause of his sexual offenses, and that she has no clear reason what made Gabriel a serial rapist. But when the casual viewer watches the episode, as there is no other tangible diagnosis to explain Gabriel's terrible actions, and Gabriel's autistic behaviors and habits are so prominent, it is easy for many watchers to latch onto the one named diagnosis, and think to themselves that whatever affected his mind, it must have had *some* effect on his crimes. The qualifier only takes up several seconds of screen time, and a distracted viewer could easily miss it.

There are several indications hinting that the prosecution has not created an entirely accurate profile of why Gabriel targets the women he does. Kibre argues to the jury that Gabriel targeted women who feared deportation, believing that they would be unwilling to go to the police. But how could he possibly have known their citizenship status? Aside from hearing the occasional accent, there is one quick clue that indicates that there is a sensory component to the way Gabriel targets his victims, as he appears to experience a level of attraction when he smells a woman passing him. This leads to the possibility that Gabriel targeted women who worked as cleaners because the lingering odors of cleaning products on their persons caused a connection to his memories of his earliest sexual experiences, which given the fact that he was a child, means that he was abused himself. No attempt is made to track down the former family employee who touched him inappropriately. The idea that his compulsive raping is connected to these sensory triggers does indicate that there could be at least some connection between his Asperger's and the separate twisted psychological influences that caused him to commit horrific acts, but the authorities never seem to make this connection. Before the verdict, Kibre notes that Gabriel showed no remorse, and she appears to believe that he has some serious mental condition that affected his behavior, but she justifies her choice not to further investigate his psyche by arguing that her job as a prosecutor is to convict rather than cure. This observation is not meant to suggest that Gabriel ought to have been placed into a mental hospital rather than a prison, and it definitely is not intended to argue that Gabriel ought not to have been punished for his crimes, but it does raise a question as to what sort of treatment people with minds like Gabriel need to receive from the criminal justice system.

A notable shared characterization about the two Aspergerian perpetrators in the early twenty-first century *Law & Order* franchise is the fact that they're portrayed as being rather pathetic. Yes, they're both highly intelligent in their respective fields, but their social awkwardness is presented in a way that makes them seem pitiable, and in the eyes of some unsympathetic people, objects of contempt and ridicule. They're both depicted as being hopeless romantically, and some characters seem surprised that Wally was able to find a wife at all, albeit temporarily. At the end of "Probability," Captain Deakins (Jamey Sheridan) quips that "they don't make criminal geniuses like they used to," implying that Wally's mental state somehow makes him a lesser figure in the captain's eyes.

Those who know Gabriel use a variety of slurs and contemptuous remarks in reference to him, ranging from the comparatively mild "eccentric" to "freak" and comparably cruel remarks. They concede he's a genius with computers, but the laughs and shaking of heads at the thought of Gabriel indicate the low esteem in which he is held by those around him. One of Gabriel's co-workers, who later sued for sexual harassment after he kept waiting for her outside of the restroom and talking about inappropriate subjects with her, declares that she initially felt sorry for him, as his clumsy attempts to chat up a woman were a miserable failure. The implication is that his demeanor and actions make it virtually impossible for him to attract a partner. Gabriel is portrayed far less sympathetically than Wally, but there's a strong implication that he is dealing with serious mental traumas that warped him in ways that the criminal justice system doesn't care to uncover. If Gabriel Duvall, an admittedly guilty man, who had immense resources at his disposal, couldn't get a favorable verdict, what chance might an autistic person of limited means, who is innocent or at least deserves the consideration of mitigating circumstances, have in court?

Wally, in particular, comes across more as a hapless victim than as an evil figure. Whether he's isolated at his desk in the basement, or when he's alone in his empty house, he has only his photographs to keep him company. Perhaps a diagnosis and therapy could have saved his marriage, but if not, having an advocate in his corner to explain his condition could have at least allowed him to remain a part of his sons' lives, as opposed to being torn apart by a uncaring family court system. It's a bleak picture of how neurotypical individuals can judge people with autism negatively, dismiss them with a negative label, and then cut them off from the connections they want to have but can't explain their desire for having. Wally didn't care about the money in itself, he cared about his family. He thought he could buy back his ex-wife's love, and as messed up as that was, it reflects how a lifetime of experiences had taught him to believe that he was unlovable, and that wealth was the only way that he could purchase affection. Wally's crimes were horrific, but at the heart of them was his desperate need for the love of his family. In itself, that challenges the declaration that people with Asperger's don't have the ability to empathize, which is mentioned in this episode. Certainly, Wally treated his sixteen victims as if they were mere abstractions, but Wally did care for his family. He just was never given the guidance he needed to show how he felt and to communicate his emotions. Viewers aren't shown any details about his wife's character or personality, so it's up to speculation why she married him in the first place and had two sons by him. Certain assumptions can be made regarding her appearance and personality, as she gained the attention of a wealthy lawyer who was willing to raise her boys, but there's no clue as to how the relationship began, or what Wally's wife's feelings were towards him at the time of the breakup of their marriage. No hint is given that either of Wally's sons inherited his mental processes. It seems as if Wally's ex-wife wanted him wiped from her life, and it's possible that the family court judge, unfamiliar with the autism spectrum, ruled unfavorably against Wally out of a biased misinterpretation of the man, and Wally and his lawyer weren't prepared to deal with this ruling.

None of this is meant to condone, excuse, or sympathize with their horrific crimes of multiple murder and serial rape. But it's obvious to the members of law enforcement who have spent time studying them that their minds are far different from the average person's. Still, there's no attempt to provide them with special accommodations in prison, which can be an even more dangerous than usual place for those with disabilities, especially those which impair interactions with other people. At Eames' suggestion, however, Goren becomes Wally's pen pal. Four years later, in "Endgame" (S6E21), Wally is shown to be surviving in prison, and Goren's infrequent letters are a source of comfort for him. To date, the character of Gabriel Duvall has not been revisited in the franchise.

In both instances, there is a strong indication that had either man been diagnosed with Asperger's at an earlier age, and provided with treatment and counselling, their lives could have been very different, and perhaps they would never have committed the crimes they did. In both cases, autism is not the core cause of their actions, but it is treated as a contributing factor.

The Brief– 'Lack of Affect' (2005)

Henry Farmer (Alan Davies) is a barrister with a crumbling personal life. Due to his out-of-control gambling habit, his wife has left him and taken custody of their son. He's now struggling to escape his massive debts, find affordable housing, and defend his clients from seemingly irrefutable criminal charges.

In "Lack of Affect," (S2E2), Dan Ottaway (Tom Burke) is in his early twenties and has a severe case of Asperger's

Syndrome. In the opening scene, he awkwardly helps a woman in the supermarket, and becomes greatly agitated. The woman thinks he's becoming violent, but fortunately his mother arrives, bearing a bright blue "Autism Alert" card, and explains her son's condition, defusing the situation. Soon afterwards, Dan's mother is found dead, and the authorities believe that Dan killed her in a fit of rage.

Dan's father Graham (Robert Pugh) is convinced his son is guilty, and tries to pressure his son to accept a plea deal for manslaughter. Dan refuses, as he's adamant he didn't do it, despite having a gap in his memory. Insisting that he doesn't tell lies, he refuses to bow to pressure to confess. Farmer discovers that Dan's father and aunt were having an affair, and that the bruises on the dead woman's body indicate that the victim had struggled with a person who wore a ring – and Dan does not wear jewelry. The prosecution seeks to introduce similar evidence to indicate that Dan had a history of violence, but the snotty teenage girl who accused Dan of attacking her is proved to be a malicious liar, who taunted Dan and called him a pedophile based on nothing but her own venom. She smugly justifies her slander by blithely stating that she thinks he looks like a child molester. It's also revealed that a psychiatrist prescribed Dan antidepressants, as he was nervous about leaving his family home for a halfway house for people with disabilities. However, he stopped taking them because he didn't like how they made him feel, and his mother started taking the pills without a doctor's supervision. One of the side effects of the pills can be erratic violent behavior.

Eventually, it's revealed that Dan's cousin Mia (Jemima Rooper) confronted Dan's mother about the affair between Dan's father and aunt, asking Dan's mother to let her husband go so Mia's mother could be happy. Addled by the medication,

Dan's mother flew into a rage, causing Mia to struggle with her aunt, leaving bruises from her engagement ring. But Mia didn't kill her. When Dan came downstairs after Mia left, Dan's mother was still in a rage and flew at her son. Instinctively, Dan put his arms around his mother in a restraining hug, the method his mother used on him when he had a meltdown. However, her struggling led to her accidental death by suffocation or asphyxiation. He blacked out the incident, believing that he couldn't have harmed his mother as he wanted her alive.

Dan is convicted of unlawful killing without intent and sentenced to two years in prison, and according to Farmer, even Dan believes that the jury came to the correct verdict. But did they really?

At the end of the episode, viewers might well ask themselves if justice had been done. Due to the defendant's Asperger's Syndrome, coupled with his utter lack of malicious intent, there is a very strong case to be made that the defendant was the victim of a justice system that was completely unequipped to deal with people whose brains were wired like his.

Dan was victimized by unfair characterization of his condition, as misconceptions about autism affect his family and almost everybody in the court. About the only people to be completely sympathetic towards Dan are Farmer, his co-counsel, and Mia. As Farmer notes at the start of the trial, the jurors are biased against Dan from the start, defining him solely by his condition and his atypical behavior. His autistic behaviors and mannerisms prejudice the jurors, and Farmer notes that they see Dan as a freak, and that any successful defense has to present him as a human being. The prosecutor seems to view Dan as an irreparably damaged freak, consistently relying on a pair of false stereotypes in order to demonize the defendant. The first is the claim that Dan's autism makes him incapable of feeling empathy, thereby slandering Dan as an emotionless murderer. The second is that people with autism are disposed towards violence, especially when they become upset. These assertions go unchallenged in court.

Even Dan's father and aunt are inclined to think the worst of him, as they both believe that he killed his mother in a fit of rage, even though they know him better than almost anybody else, and know that he has never committed a deliberate act of physical harm. While it's never explicitly spelled out, their conclusions may be influenced by selfish wishful thinking. If Dan were locked away in prison for an extended period of time, he'd be out of their hair. There's a strong implication that they *want* him to be guilty, as his crime and conviction would eliminate two problems at once– the ending of the marriage and the removal of the need to look over a son with special needs.

Once again, this is a case where an autistic person is smeared for lack of empathy, selfishness, and violence by neurotypical people who are even more guilty of the aforementioned callous behaviors. Dan's father and aunt were having a secret affair, and Dan's father was planning to leave his wife. Dan's cousin wanted her aunt and uncle's marriage broken up with no concern over what it might mean for Dan and his mother. Dan's mother was planning a trip away with her husband once Dan moved into the halfway home, so just as she thought she'd get a second lease on her marriage, her husband was about to shatter her life. The teenaged girl who falsely claimed Dan was a pedophile gets off with no punishment whatsoever – no slander charges, not even a charge for mistreatment of a disabled person. Once again, the neurotypical people are the ones who demonstrate a shocking lack of empathy and compassion, but it is the person with autism who is branded as an emotionless monster.

What's frustrating is that Dan's autism is only ever used against him, painting him as a monster who is perfectly capable of killing his own mother without a trace of remorse. Farmer's defense revolves around total innocence. However, once it's revealed that Dan caused his mother's death purely by accident after she attacked him in a medication-fueled rage, everybody, even Dan, accepts that he must bear responsibility for his mother's death. But why? Looking at the facts, Dan's mother took unprescribed antidepressants that made her violent. She attacked Dan. Surely a plea of self-defense could be in order, especially since there is a question as to how well he could understand the true magnitude of the threat. Not only that, but the possibility of mitigation due to his autistic mental state is never put forward. There is a strong case that Dan is completely guiltless. His own feeling that he should be punished is due to his horror over remembering what he did, but he is probably being much too hard on himself. In addition, why is Dan in prison? He's been left bruised and battered by other inmates while in custody previously. Given his condition, he's not safe in a jail with violent inmates. Even if he were to serve time, he should be in a secure mental health facility where he can get proper care and protection. This verdict and sentence is a tragedy, and Farmer is at fault for failing to look after the best interests of his client by pursuing all available lines of defense.

The final scene between Dan and his father shows an incarcerated Dan adjusting surprisingly well to prison life, which seems unlikely and a little pat due to his past difficulty adjusting to new surroundings, strangers, and noises. He actually expresses a desire to stay even longer, as he's in the process of reorganizing the prison library, and he doesn't think that two years is enough time to complete the job. The closing exchange is meant to be touching, as father and son reenact a scene from *E.T.*, calling back to Dan's father's previous comment about calling his son "E.T." growing up, as the autistic boy seemed like a little alien to him. Though the dialogue is played to make Dan's father seem sympathetic for not having the emotional connection he wanted with his son, on examination the comment is rather cruel, especially as Dan demonstrates that he was aware of the nickname and has embraced it without realizing the offensive connotations. The final message is that Dan's trouble understanding emotions really does make him an alien, an outsider different from most of society, and therefore a less sympathetic character who deserves to be punished for an accident resulting from a situation he could not predict, control, nor understand.

    It is an unsatisfying ending to a promising premise, and it rings emotionally and intellectually hollow. It's not the fault of Tom Burke, who gives a sensitive and tragic performance. It is the rush to blame Dan, treating his condition as an irreparable flaw, when in fact it's those around him who bear more culpability. Over twenty years, none of his doctors or caregivers devised an effective system to help him understand emotions or connections, aside from a book of pictures with words describing the emotions shown. His psychiatrist prescribed him antidepressants with serious side effects, never realizing that the differences in autistic brain chemistry might cause medications to affect Dan differently than they would a neurotypical person. Once again, Dan's mother took his antidepressants without a doctor's supervision, and the result was erratic and violent behavior that badly agitated Dan. His father and aunt were having an affair, and it's implied that his aunt wanted him locked away for a long stretch of time so he'd be out of her hair. The prosecutor callously equated autism with absence of empathy and violence, and the jurors couldn't look past the disability. Not only that, but his lawyer failed to pursue legitimate defenses. "Lack of Affect" falls flat due to its failure to call out neurotypical people and the criminal justice system for their unfair treatment of the autistic, and it pronounces a sentence upon poor Dan that is both unmerited and inhumane. The title "Lack of Affect" may be intended to refer to Dan's manner of speaking and emoting, but there's a second meaning to the phrase. It could be interpreted as a reference to the fact that the Dan's pain and struggling did not affect the minds of the jury and the court. In *The Brief*, the justice system can't or won't help Dan, but it will punish him. And what happens when he's released? Will his father care for him, or will his dad focus on his new relationship, leaving Dan to be shipped off to the halfway house for people like him, forever branded as a mother-killer and treated with suspicion by all? *The Brief* tries for a happy ending, but what it presents is a young man with serious disabilities who has been chewed up and spat out by an unfeeling court and self-absorbed relatives.

L-Death Note Monster Speech

In all iterations of *Death Note*, L acts as if he is above the law. He often commits crimes in order to achieve his objectives, but in each case, the infractions are strictly for the purpose of catching Kira. For the purposes of this section and simplicity, only the anime version will be addressed. While the official police are restricted in their actions, bound to rules, regulations, and warrants, L has no such restrictions and no scruples against violating Japanese law in order to pursue his investigative objectives. Having massive monetary reserves and the ability to convince the governments of the world to acquiesce to his requests for assistance, at least most of the time, L isn't bound by laws, and frequently adopts an "ends justify the means" approach to his investigations.

Throughout the anime series, L violates Japanese law. Among his most notable transgressions, he places a death row inmate in mortal peril in order to test Kira's powers; he installs illegal video surveillance cameras; he pickpockets a phone; and he detains a suspect without legal authorization, keeping her for weeks in a position that could very well be defined as torturous. At no point does L feel any guilt for his actions, even when Chief Soichiro Yagami raises concerns about the morality of his actions. L never appears to derive any pleasure from breaking rules, as his only concern is to win the battle of wits by obtaining the evidence to identify and stop Kira. Personal benefit is irrelevant to him, aside from the personal satisfaction of victory. L acts as a vigilante, breaking whatever laws stand in his way of solving the case. He has no fear of legal reprisals, knowing that with his reputation and influence, he almost certainly will never be charged for any crime. Additionally, given the supernatural aspect of the case, a strong argument could be made that extraordinary measures are necessary in order to address a situation that cannot be properly investigate through traditional means, and extensive steps must be taken to protect L and *his* allies from possible magical reprisals. In L's mind, his abilities and righteousness mean that the rules don't apply to him… although at some points, it seems as if L has a far more negative self-image.

Of course, breaking the rules is often par for the course on crime shows, where rebel police officers and antiestablishment private detectives are always playing fast and loose in order to achieve their goals. L certainly isn't the first or only detective to perform illegal searches or surveillance, or to put someone else in mortal danger in order to advance a case. Plenty of neurotypical detectives do exactly the same thing. But L is aware of how his mind differentiates him from most people, not just in terms of his advanced intelligence, but in his ability to connect with others and engage in many aspects of life.

The anime of *Death Note* has a pair of companion pieces, punningly titled *Relight*. In this pair of feature-length movies, the anime has been heavily abridged, with most of the subplots deleted, entire storylines collapsed, and additional scenes added. Some of these new scenes change details about the narrative, such as a new meeting between L and Light, and some added scenes enhance characterization. *Death Note: Relight– L's Successors*, the second part of this condensation, features a flashback scene not present in the original anime, where L speaks through a laptop to a group of children at the orphanage where he was once raised. When asked what scares him, L replies "monsters," and elaborates in a telling monologue.

> "There are many types of monsters in this world. Monsters who will not show themselves and who cause trouble, monsters who abduct children, monsters who devour dreams, monsters who suck blood... and... monsters who always tell lies. Lying monsters are a real nuisance. They are much more cunning than other monsters. They pose as humans even though they have no understanding of the human heart; they eat even though they've never experienced hunger; they study even though they have no interest in academics; they seek friendship even though they do not know how to love. If I were to encounter such a monster, I would likely be eaten by it. Because in truth, I am that monster."

It's an intense and telling monologue, that reflects L's level of self-awareness as to his own mind and habits, but it is also overly harsh. As Dan on *The Brief* seemed to accept his designation as an alien, L feels that it's accurate to call himself a monster. The lies he tells aren't just untruths told to solve a case. They reflect his inability to understand how others feel and think, and so he goes through the motions, mimicking mannerisms that other people do, all in an attempt to appear more like everybody else. It's a common feeling amongst people with autism that there's something "broken," or "off" about them, simply because how they are wired prevents them from forming the connections and understandings that other people do – or at least, to the extent that they *believe* other people are able to feel and empathize. The Temperance Brennan refrain of "I don't get it" doesn't just apply to the occasional joke. It can refer to the reasons for social niceties or reacting to conventions.

Tellingly, unlike Light, L never thought his supremely intelligent mind made him an *ubermensch*, innately superior to others. On the contrary, he focused on what he lacked– the ability to connect and understand others at the level he thought normal. As a result, he saw himself as subhuman… a monster. This is L's cautionary tale– if someone doesn't learn how to understand why his mind works the way it does, the frustration may turn inward, turning to disgusted self-loathing. There was no one to reframe L's mindset by diagnosing autism, revealing that he wasn't monstrous, just wired differently. No one, not even Watari, was there to affirm L's basic humanity. Instead of viewing himself as simply the possessor of a different kind of mind, L saw himself as a deformed creature.

And so, autism can cause a great gulf between an affected individual and the rest of humanity, as a constant feeling of being unable to understand creates an unscalable wall, a feeling exacerbated by self-flagellating thoughts that one is a freak, an alien, or a monster. L never learned how to develop connections with others, but did anybody ever try to help him? L was fully aware of his problems, and instead of trying to understand or overcome his issues with connection, he chose to internalize them as an inherent and inescapable flaw, and this caused him to doubt his own humanity, with his acceptance the self-loathing description of himself as a monster.

Zack Addy – Bones

From the series' pilot up to the final episode of *Bones'* third season, Zack Addy (Eric Millegan) is an amiable, likable, awkward member of the team. As Dr. Brennan's graduate student, he was personally chosen to study with her, and she soon came to care for him as a little brother. For his part, Zack often seemed to have an unrequited crush on Bones. Zack was an effective and much-liked member of the detecting team, whose work was often critical to solving cases, and some of his co-workers were his best friends. That all changes in Season Three finale "The Pain in the Heart," (S3E15). Over the course of the season, the team hunts The Gormogon, a serial killer with cannibalistic tendencies who leaves behind bone-related clues and works with an apprentice.

In "The Pain in the Heart," Zack is initially a figure of sympathy after an explosion during an experiment seriously injures his hands. After Bones discovers that Zack made deliberate mistakes in his previous analysis of the Gormogon case, she deduces that Zack is the Gormogon's apprentice.

When Bones confronts Zack in the hospital, he confesses without much prompting to the murder of a lobbyist earlier in the season. Though the details are hazy, the Gormogon was apparently able to brainwash Zack into becoming his assistant. Showing no anger and an uncharacteristic amount of affection, Bones swiftly deprograms him, and Zack reveals the Gormogon's location, where the multiple murderer is killed in a fight by authorities. Zack takes a plea deal, and goes to a mental hospital for life for the murder.

Zack only makes a couple of appearances over the next couple of seasons, and goes completely absent from the show for several years, but in one of his early guest appearances, he explains to the psychologist, Sweets, that he did not commit the actual crime, but was only an accessory. Towards the end of the series run, after Zack has spent nearly a decade in an asylum, Bones and the rest of the team re-investigate the case, prove Zack did not physically kill anybody and was psychologically manipulated by the Gormogon, and earn his release.

Sherlock – "His Last Vow"

The climactic scene of "His Last Vow" is a very controversial one for Holmesians. On Christmas Day, Sherlock and John attempt to negotiate with the power-hungry blackmailer Charles Augustus Magnussen (Lars Mikkelsen) at his palatial home. Magnussen has evidence that can expose the dark past of John's wife, Mary (Amanda Abbington), and Sherlock's titular vow to protect the couple and their unborn child leads him to take extraordinary steps. An attempt to use Mycroft's (Mark Gatiss) confidential information-filled laptop as the bait to justify an official search is thwarted when Magnussen revealed that he does not keep his blackmail evidence on the premises, and instead commits everything to memory. When government agents prepare to storm the property, Magnussen smugly taunts the pair, believing that they're the ones who will face the consequences of the law, not him. To save Mary and all of Magnussen's other victims, Holmes grabs a gun and kills Magnussen.

Turning to violence is a seemingly uncharacteristic stratagem for a character who's known for utilizing his intelligence to untangle seemingly insoluble problems. There were certainly other options that could have prevented Holmes from using a gun to resolve the situation. As the closing scenes indicate, Sherlock knew that he very likely had an out from the situation, as his brother Mycroft would most likely use his influence to save him from serious punishment.

There were perhaps other options that could at least have placed Magnussen in check if not outright defeated him. False evidence could have been crafted to incriminate Magnussen and then counter-blackmail him into remaining silent, or a false story (or even better, a series of stories) could have been released with Magnussen's imprimatur in order to discredit him. Release one provably false story, and the blackmailer loses his power, as no one will believe him when he attempts to publicize an embarrassing truth. This is the strategy Hercule Poirot used in Agatha Christie's *The Labours of Hercules*, and though not as dramatic an offensive, it's certainly much more morally and legally unobjectionable. Indeed, all Sherlock has to do is hand Mycroft the laptop and whisper in his ear, and Mycroft can declare that the laptop was wiped or encoded in such a way that no information could possibly have been leaked to Magnussen, so Sherlock and John cannot be charged with any crime, giving the pair more time to launch a counter-attack on the media magnate.

Notably, Sherlock reaffirms his "high-functioning sociopath" self-diagnosis right before firing the gun, even though this description seems less accurate with each passing episode. Why say this? Is it to put a bit of fear into Magnussen's last moments, to let the blackmailer realize that his opponent has no compunction about using methods most people would find objectionable? Or is it an attempt to convince *himself* that he will feel nothing after pulling the trigger, a means of anesthetizing himself to the pangs of conscience that might be forthcoming?

There is another way to interpret Sherlock's violent actions. As Magnussen waits for Mycroft's team of mercenaries to arrive, he delightedly humiliates John by flicking his face. John stands there, seemingly accepting the mortification in order to protect his wife, but his posture is rigid and the anger is building in his face, reminiscent of a couple of episodes earlier, as John was working up a slow boil in response to Sherlock's reveal that he was still alive and had kept John in the dark, leading to a physical brawl between the two friends. When one starts to suspect that John was just seconds away from snapping and attacking Magnussen, this puts a different complexion on Sherlock's actions. Sherlock saw his friend seething and knew that a violent outburst was likely. Knowing that John could lurch forward at any moment and snap Magnussen's neck, Sherlock struck first to prevent John from killing Magnussen. Not only did he not want the guilt of this homicide on his friend's conscience, but Sherlock knew that Mycroft would be far less likely to protect John than his own brother.

Will Graham – Hannibal

Over the course of *Hannibal's* three seasons, all of the characters are drawn deeper into a world filled with evil and grotesque violence. Not only do already homicidal and brutal characters grow even more twisted over time, but even those working with the FBI to catch killers (save for a couple of amiable laboratory technicians) commit acts that they would never believe themselves capable of committing at the start of the series. Will Graham, who feared losing himself if he returned to work placing himself in the minds of criminals, was right to be concerned. The television series goes far deeper into the darkest regions of Graham's psyche than the novel *Red Dragon* or the two earlier adaptations, and Will crosses lines that he never even approached in the original source material.

Initially, Will begins psychiatric counseling with Hannibal Lecter (Mads Mikkelsen) after he's compelled to shoot a serial killer in the series premiere. This volatile situation was surreptitiously sparked by a phone call from Lecter, who warned the killer of Will's impending arrival as a means of seeing what might happen next. The killing was a justified shoot, but taking a man's life, even if it was necessary to save another person, affects Will's psyche deeply. Most disturbing to Will is the possibility that he derived a certain level of satisfaction, even pleasure, from the kill. Will's gift to replicate a murderer's mind is a dangerous tool, as he starts worrying if one day he will mirror a homicidal maniac's psyche in his own brain, and be unable to banish it. He picked exactly the wrong psychiatrist, as Lecter delights in setting up situations where people are forced to kill, and then exploring how the fatal act affects them afterwards.

Most of Will's legal transgressions take place in season two, where he is falsely imprisoned for Lecter's crimes. At one point, Will sends another serial killer who admires Will's supposed slaying after Lecter. This is a pivotal moment for Will, as he is essentially ordering a murder for hire. He might be able to justify it by pointing out that he's saving Lecter's future victims, but really, his primary motivation is revenge. The attempt fails, but the stain remains on Will's soul, and his colleagues at the FBI are aware of what he's done, and are even more convinced of his dangerous madness. Upon regaining his freedom, he's determined to convince the authorities of Lecter's guilt, and to do so, he has to go into some disturbing and dark places. After Lecter sends a murderer to attack Will, Will is forced to kill his assailant in self-defense, which causes a *rapprochement* between the two men, as Lecter now considers them even. To further convince Lecter that he has gone to the dark side, Will poses the corpse in a grisly tableau like Lecter does with his victims, and later pretends to kill the reporter Freddie Lounds and gives Lecter a piece of flesh– ostensibly from Lounds– for Lecter to prepare into a meal they can share. Like many undercover officers, Will has to do some unpleasant actions to win the trust of his target, but while most law enforcement officials in such a position do so with the approval of their bosses, Will only has the tacit support of Jack Crawford, and the higher-ups at the FBI do not approve of his actions. By the end of season two, Will breaks down and warns Lecter, compromising the mission and giving Lecter a chance to escape, though the situation does not unfold as planned.

    Does Will's supposed autism have any effect on driving his criminal actions? It's reportedly asserted that his mind is uniquely designed to see into criminals' brains, but in this case, Will is obsessed with catching Lecter. Is this obsessive single-mindedness connected to autism? It's impossible to make a definitive statement. Will is aware that the more time he spends profiling murderers, the harder it is to retreat in to a happier, more peaceful mental state. If Will really does feel "hyper-empathy" like the show's creator Bryan Fuller suggests, then in practice, his focus on his target leads him to be blinded to the needs and wellbeing of other, innocent people who may be caught in the fray. It's hazardous to attribute any of Will's actions to an autistic mindset, since the diagnosis within the show comes from Will himself, and outside the show comes from Fuller's non-clinical dramatization of how he thinks a mind on the spectrum may work, and may overlook numerous other psychological factors that may argue against an autism diagnosis. As for Will's protection of Lecter, could any of it be connected with the fact that he believes that Lecter is the only person in the world who truly understands his mind?

Professor T – "The Family"

In "The Family," (S2E3), Professor T must uncover the truth behind the deaths of a family of four. All of the members of the family are found lined up on the living room couch, and each succumbed to a different cause of death. The father died of carbon monoxide poisoning, the mother swallowed an overdose of pills and alcohol, the daughter died of a broken neck, and the son succumbed from inhaling too much natural gas. The son had autism and was hypersensitive to sounds and other stimuli. His need for constant attention and care annoyed his neurotypical sister. She resented his complaining about her guitar playing and envied all of the support her brother got from their father. In the flashback scenes (which are possibly not an accurate depiction of the past, but instead are simply Professor T's biased personal reconstructions of events), the sister shows no understanding or compassion towards her brother. She is only thinking about how she is affected.

One clue that needs explanation is the fact that the daughter's guitar was smashed. After running through the possibilities, Professor T analyzes the crime scene and deduces the following series of events. The professor believes that the father and daughter got into an argument over her music playing, and as a result the father grabbed his daughter's guitar and smashed it. Professor T suggests that the father had undiagnosed autism, though a much milder form than his son. This is due to the father's obsessive cleaning and ordering of the house, along with his meltdown in front of a co-worker that led to the downward spiral of his career. When Professor T makes his diagnosis, his audience of police officers looks at each other, as if to say, "It takes one to know one," silently referencing the professor's own undiagnosed and never officially admitted autism.

In the professor's reconstruction, the daughter stormed away from her father, and caught her toe on the one out-of-place item in the house: a slight peeling of the carpet at the top of the stairs. She caught her toe in it and fell down the stairwell, breaking her neck in the process. Her father was devastated, and feared not just going to prison himself, but the affect his absence would have on his son. He hypothesizes that the father arranged his daughter's body neatly on the couch. Initially he planned to commit suicide by gassing himself in the kitchen, but he decided that death was a preferable option for his son than living without his care. So the father picked up his son from his group session, and drove him home, neglecting to turn off the stove. When they arrived home, the father ran the car in the closed garage, planning to asphyxiate them both. He made no attempt to restrain his son, he simply believed the autistic teen would sit quietly in the car and allow himself to be poisoned. Of course, the son wanted to live, and he forced his way out of the car and into the house, which was directly connected to the garage. Apparently the son was perfectly capable of movement, but the father was already too overcome to budge, so he remained in the car and died soon afterwards. Unfortunately for the son, he ran straight into the gas-filled kitchen, which apparently was so toxic that he collapsed to the ground before he could flee outside, turn off the oven, or even open a window. The mother came home to find her whole family dead, somehow managing not to fall victim to either the car exhaust or the gas oven fumes that knocked out her husband and son in seconds. After airing the house and garage out long enough that the police only detected faint whiffs of gas odors, she dragged her son and husband to the couch, and then sat beside her loved ones, consumed a massive dose of pills and alcohol and died.

It's a seemingly tidy solution, but the two different gases conveniently affecting people at different rates, plus the fact that the meticulous husband just happened to overlook the two points in the house that killed both his children, call Professor T's solution into question. After closer review, the solution is sloppy, both in terms of logic and in its clumsy treatment of autism. The son clearly has serious difficulties connected to his autism, but he's not utterly helpless. For the father to believe that death is the best option for him isn't a loving act, but rather the twisted, controlling act of a family annihilator, a narcissist who believes his son can't survive without him. In this episode, the two dead people with autism (or at least, one of whom allegedly has autism, based solely on the theories of Professor T, who is not a licensed psychologist and never met any of the people he's describing) embody a deeply negative portrayal of the condition, and oversimplify the challenges that go into a proper diagnosis. The son is treated as hypersensitive and unable to either function when exposed to distracting stimuli, nor explain his reactions in a manner that will make peace with his sister. Was soundproofing a room or even giving the son noise-cancelling headphones never considered? The autistic son is essentially a one-dimensional victim, a character who is treated as needing attention and assistance to survive, and no effort is made to suggest that he could take care of himself. Perhaps he couldn't, but the portrayal in the show presents him as utterly helpless, aside from managing to save himself from the gas-filled garage before falling victim to a second poisonous room. Professor T's statement that the deaths weren't murders is puzzling. According to his theory, there were two suicides and one accident, but the son's death was indeed a murder, unless the professor means that since the father "accidentally" failed to turn off the gas oven during his first suicide attempt, it should count as an accident, but legally and morally, the father murdered his son.

  As for the father, his actions can be viewed as monstrous. His daughter's death was an accident, but his plan to kill his son, leaving them all for his wife to find her entire family gone without so much as a note of explanation… to blame all of this as an autistic inability to understand how to respond to a situation or to expect how people would respond, strains credulity. Perhaps he was influenced by his passionately euthanasia-supporting wife, who promoted death as the solution to problems. Even if one accepts the father's behavior as a combination of overreaction and emotional blindness shaped by autism, it's one of the most negative portrayals of an autistic mind discussed in this book. The father is a sick, selfish man, and the son is portrayed as little more than a simple victim. Compared to the quiet, restrained struggles of Professor T's own undiagnosed autism, the picture created of the deceased father and son's autism is a crude caricature devoid of nuance.

Dexter Morgan – Dexter

Dexter Morgan is famous for being a serial killer who only murders other killers, hiding his deadly activities while performing a respectable day job as a blood spatter analyst for the Miami Police Department. As stated earlier, Dexter's psyche is far more complex than a single diagnosis of sociopathy, it is possible that autism may or may not be one of the factors that shape his twisted psyche.

The question that follows is, to what extent does autism affect his murders? It has been earlier established that there is absolutely no known link between autism and criminality. Certainly, sticking to set routines can be autism-influenced, and Dexter notes how fond he is of his rituals, though as the series progresses he becomes more willing to change up his traditional habits in order to protect himself when he realizes that his rituals may eventually prove incriminating. For example, he famously takes a drop of blood after slicing his victim's cheek right before the murder, and then preserves it in a glass slide and keeps it in a box. Even after the slide box is discovered by an antagonist and eventually winds up in the hands of the authorities, Dexter buys a new box soon afterwards and continues this ritual until seasons seven, when he realizes that taking trophies from his victims is just too dangerous for him.

His attention to detail may also be a factor in the care he takes in preparing his "murder rooms," usually lining the walls of an isolated place with plastic wrap in order to make for complete and easy cleanup. With a perhaps uncharacteristic amount of self-introspection, he notes, "I am a very neat monster." A form of OCD could be an influence on Dexter as well, but once again, all of these potential diagnoses are purely theoretical. Trauma and antisocial personality disorder may give him the urge to kill, but any possible autism in Dexter's psyche has a far more notable effect on his personal life, particularly the problems he has understanding and replicating emotions and interacting with others.

Choi Sang-hyeon – Extraordinary Attorney Woo

At the end of the penultimate episode of *Extraordinary Attorney Woo's* first season, the viewers are provided with the surprise reveal of Choi Sang-hyeon (Choi Hyun-jin), Woo Young-Woo's half-brother on her mother's side. Choi Sang-hyeon is also an autistic savant. Although he is only a high-schooler, he has an advanced talent with computer programming and has won many awards for his cybersecurity projects. He's uncomfortable looking people in the eye when he talks to them, preferring to look downwards. Rubik's Cubes are a favorite toy of his, and he has many of them, as well as an alarm clock and a flash drive with Rubik's Cube patterns on them. Though he doesn't explain the point explicitly, playing with a Rubik's Cube seems to be a calming influence on him.

Choi Sang-hyeon comes into Woo Young-Woo's life after he realizes that he has inadvertently been drawn into a high-stakes game of corporate skullduggery. Kim Chan-hong (Ryu Kyung-hwan) recruited Choi Sang-hyeon to breach his company's online security, presumably to send a message that better precautions needed to be taken. When Choi Sang-hyeon hacked into the company's systems, he was not being malicious. Charitably, he might be considered naïve, being influenced by the company's head, who had befriended Choi Sang-hyeon as a mentor. He had no desire to harm anybody.

What's notable is the level of integrity Choi Sang-hyeon demonstrates when he's dealing with the fallout of his hacking. All he had to do was stay silent, and it's unlikely that anybody would have learned of his involvement. After he confessed to his mother, his only present parent told him to keep quiet, as she feared that a scandal could crush her political ambitions. Choi Sang-hyeon refused to remain silent, and turned to his half-sister for help.

A simple lie could have shielded Choi Sang-hyeon from potential legal repercussions. All he would have had to say is that he was hired as a "white hat" hacker to test the security of the system, being told that he wasn't accessing actual confidential client information, but instead was just testing the system to find weaknesses, and then realized the truth after he had completed the task. Certainly no one could disprove that. He could have been chastised for being credulous, but if he'd just lied and said that he'd initially believed his actions were part of a necessary security test that endangered no one's privacy, that story could have provided a strong defense against legal repercussions.

Perhaps this little self-protecting fib simply never occurred to Choi Sang-hyeon. However, there is much to suggest that Choi Sang-hyeon is an extremely honest person, bolstering the trope that suggests that people on the autism spectrum often have extreme trouble saying anything that is not the purest truth. On more than one occasion, Choi Sang-hyeon voices his disapproval of wealthy families who use their money and influence to protect their spoiled, transgressing progeny from the consequences of their wrongdoing. Such people seem to upset Choi Sang-hyeon deeply, and he is determined not to be one of them. In addition to his commitment to honesty, Choi Sang-hyeon embodies the commonly cited characteristic of people with autism holding both themselves and others to high moral standards. Having inadvertently committed a crime, Choi Sang-hyeon films a confession and gives it to Woo Young-Woo to use as evidence, and berates his mother for trying to cover up his misdeeds in order to protect her own political ambitions. For Choi Sang-hyeon, the path forward is clear – state the truth whatever the consequences, apologize to anybody who has been hurt by fears over breached data, and accept what comes as a result of making the situation right. Like Wally Stevens, Choi Sang-hyeon does not believe that he deserves a "get out of jail free card," but unlike Wally, Choi Sang-hyeon was prompted to reveal the truth at a time when no one had any suspicions of his involvement. Doing the crime means doing time, or at least some form of retribution. Choi Sang-hyeon comes across as a basically good person who was manipulated into a situation where he didn't realize the seriousness and illegality of his consequences until afterwards.

Concluding Reflections

Ultimately, it's the creative works that people can debate without resolution that stick with them the longest. Studying these autistic perpetrators leads to many unanswered questions. Of the characters discussed here, all except for Dan Ottaway made a conscious decision to commit crimes (or at least morally dubious acts), though they bear widely varying degrees of guilt. Choi Sang-hyeon, for example, may be more of a dupe than anything else. Should autism be treated as a mitigating factor in criminal cases, at least in some cases? Is the portrayal of an empathy-free autistic person in some of the aforementioned cases a stereotype based on an incomplete understanding of autism? Was it autism that made the characters described here commit criminal acts, or was it other factors, ranging from exigent circumstances to other mental factors, that shaped them? These are questions that are left unexplored by the shows, and are left to the viewers to analyze.

Some of the characters discussed became criminals deliberately for some sort of personal gain, others by accident, while others acted in the pursuit of justice. In popular culture, for many people with or without autism, justice can become an obsession that can go too far. All of these perpetrators here focused on one goal at the expense of broader issues such as morality and adherence to the law. Ultimately, these dramatizations of autism often hint that the minds of the perpetrators played roles in their decisions, but these shows generally fail to explore thoroughly the impact of the character's mind on the criminal actions being committed.

CHAPTER ELEVEN
Looking Through an Autistic Lens

For years, autism advocates have argued that while autism may qualify as a disability, an autistic mind is not inherently inferior to a neurotypical mind, and to expect that all brains should function in the same way is prejudiced and unrealistic. In many of the series shown here, the autistic sleuths are criticized, denigrated, mocked, or chided for their actions and behaviors, which are clearly influenced by their mental processes. In many cases, the message is implicit: The person with autism needs to adjust in order to fit in better, or that the autistic person needs to learn how to treat others better. The autistic person must learn how to be more "normal."

But what if this perspective simply is not fair? What if the autistic person, despite having trouble understanding how to function socially, is being targeted simply for being different? What if the people telling the autistic person to change are setting unfair expectations, and perhaps overlooking worse transgressions in others? If this is the case, then viewers need to refocus how they view these characters, and in order to do so, their characters need to be defended, partly through looking at them through their own point of view, or at least a perspective that is determined to take their sides.

In order to explain how a sympathetic autism lens can reshape how we understand these characters, a few of the most frequently criticized and maligned autistic sleuths will be profiled here: Cumberbatch's Sherlock, Doc Martin, and Christopher Boone.

Of all the detectives in this study, Cumberbatch's Sherlock is probably the most criticized for his social behaviors. When critics and viewers try to sum up the Cumberbatch Sherlock's personality, he's generally considered at best insensitive to others, and at a worse, a total jerk. Especially early in the series, he's aggressive in his denigration of others, asserting his intellectual superiority, and occasionally humiliating others through making public observations that his targets would rather keep private.

In *Sherlock's* first episode, "A Study in Pink," (S1E1) Sherlock treats members of the official police with disdain, famously defusing their accusation of psychopathy with his own self-diagnosis of high-functioning sociopathy, served with a generous helping of derision. Viewed casually, it's easy and common to view Sherlock as the unpleasant one here, a man so arrogant and certain of his own mental superiority that he cannot be bothered to show a modicum of respect to those he sees as lesser beings.

But if one watches those early scenes in "A Study in Pink" with a predisposition to take Sherlock's side, one can view his comments as not merely offensive (in all senses of the term), but *defensive* tactics meant to protect himself from bullying and slander. Lestrade (Rupert Graves) knows he needs Sherlock's help, but it's Philip Anderson (Jonathan Aris) and Sgt. Sally Donovan (Vinette Robinson) who view Sherlock with utter disgust and contempt. They show no respect for Sherlock's powers of observation and induction, and instead treat him as a freak, and Donovan describes him to John as an unwanted interloper who is on the cusp of madness and destruction. Her evidence for their dim view of Sherlock's future? There doesn't appear to be any, other than her own gut feelings, and potentially, her wounded pride at having a layman called in to assist in solving a case. Clearly, Anderson and Donovan have been acquainted with Sherlock for quite some time, and this open hostility has almost certainly been going for a while. Their dislike of Sherlock seems fairly visceral, and though the cause of this negativity must to a certain extent be theoretical, it seems likely that jealousy and resentment towards Sherlock's enhanced powers are connected to the feelings of inferiority that arise when they compare themselves to him. When Sherlock exposes the affair between Anderson (who is married) and Donovan in a way that is both subtle and devastating, it might be viewed as a retaliatory measure, used to defuse the situation and allow Sherlock to retrieve his dignity from the people who seek to humiliate him.

By the end of the final episode of the second series, "The Reichenbach Fall" (S2E3), Anderson and Donovan have swallowed Moriarty's lies whole, and are leading the charge to have Sherlock discredited as a fraud. By the mini-episode linking series two and three, "Many Happy Returns," (S3E0), Anderson has lost his marriage and his job, and he is wracked with guilt with the belief that his promotion of a lie ruined Sherlock's reputation and presumably drove him to suicide, but Anderson is saved from total despair by his belief that Sherlock is still alive. When series three's first full episode, "The Empty Hearse" (S3E1) opens, Sherlock's name has been completely cleared, and Anderson devotes most of his spare time to celebrating Sherlock's life and career, becoming both a rather pathetic figure and almost affectionate parody of *Sherlock's* real-life avid fans. Though Anderson is never shown to have gotten his life back on track, he has redeemed his former nasty unpleasantness by his constant attempts to make amends.

Donovan, in contrast, never says so much as "sorry" for her part at smearing Sherlock's name, and shows no remorse for her supposed contribution to provoking a man to suicide, especially when it is later proven than he was wrongly accused. Donovan's screen time is fairly marginal, but in nearly all of her appearances, save for her brief cameo in "The Sign of Three"

(S3E2), where she appears to be doing a reasonably competent job assisting Lestrade, the lion's share of her lines are spent denigrating and disliking Holmes.

Over the course of her handful of appearances, Donovan has an affair with Anderson. She is unable to match Holmes's detecting skills, and instead of attempting to improve her own abilities, she attempts to tear Holmes down by spreading rumors about his mental instability and potential violent tendencies. The moment there's a chance to denounce Sherlock as a duplicitous criminal, she goes all in to promote this theory without doing a scrap of detective work to confirm the validity of the allegations. When her former lover is crushed at their target's suicide, she isn't shown to have any guilt whatsoever. To be fair, Donovan isn't shown much at all, but she's still able to pursue her career without any known repercussions for a high-profile false accusation. In summary, Donovan's entire role in the series revolves around cheating, spreading defamation of character, and targeting a professional rival through a vendetta where she exploits her position in law enforcement to target an innocent man. All this, and she isn't shown to have even the slightest moral twinge at her own behavior. Who's the "high-functioning sociopath" *now*?

Moving away from Anderson and Donovan, Sherlock is often castigated for his treatment of Molly Hooper. From their first appearance in "A Study in Pink" (S1E1), Molly is attracted to Sherlock. She puts on lipstick, she asks him out to coffee, and then she feels hurt when he fails to respond with romantic overtures of his own. He notices the lipstick but doesn't express attraction, and the offer of coffee is seen simply as a means of refreshment rather than as a social interaction, ideally a prelude as to something more. Throughout the series, viewers are regularly guided to think "Poor Molly," as a heartsick woman's feelings are continually trod upon by an insensitive clod. Certainly Molly isn't at fault here, but if an attempt is made to see their interactions through an autistic lens, neither is Sherlock.

Blaming Sherlock for his ineptitude at reading Molly's signs is the result of looking at him with neurotypical expectations. Social cues and navigating the world of dating are challenging enough for most people. They can be close to impossible for people on the autism spectrum. Before moving forward, it is crucial to reframe Sherlock's behavior towards Molly. First, let it be assumed that any hurt Sherlock inflicts on Molly feelings is *unintentional*. Second, viewers need to proceed on the assumption that whatever Sherlock's aptitude in applying his powers of observation to solving crimes and pursuing other intellectual endeavors and applying his powers, when it comes to romantic situations and understanding other people's wants and needs, Sherlock is laboring at a disadvantage.

If we view Cumberbatch's Sherlock through a sympathetic autistic lens, it may be concluded that his seeming brusqueness and insensitivity are not merely an unfeeling lack of empathy, but are rather a form of armor against a mocking and suspicious world. Sherlock is different. He's not inherently cruel or sociopathic, but he has built up his defenses after a lifetime of mockery and ostracization, and his seemingly rude behaviors are a mixture of pushing others away as a means of self-defense that has gone beyond his control, and his inherent neurological difficulties in understanding the feelings of others.

Moving on to *Doc Martin*, the title character has always been known for his prickly personality. Though he possesses extensive medical knowledge, which combined with his thoroughness and observational skills, make him an excellent medical detective, his bedside manner is gruff at best, and his poor social skills affect his personal relationships in widely varying ways. His peers in the medical profession tend to treat him as an annoying oddity, a brilliant mind whose personality is so abrasive that they are reluctant to assist him in rebuilding his career or even hold a conversation with him. In contrast, the villagers of Portwenn mostly take the doctor's surliness in stride, shrugging off any perceived slights and rarely taking offense. Despite his curtness, the supporting cast all like the doctor and respect his medical abilities.

The one major character who is deeply frustrated by the doctor's difficulty with emotions and connections is his eventual wife, Louisa. Martin's challenges with interactions have a debilitating effect on his married life, mostly in the early years of their marriage. Over the course of the seventh series, Martin and Louisa go for couples counselling

There are, of course, at least two sides to every marital argument, but in this case, the lack of an autism diagnosis binds Martin's hands and prevents him from both defending himself or improving his marriage. Louisa's main complaint in the marriage is that she feels that she is not receiving the level of emotional support she wants or needs. This is certainly not an unreasonable request, but in a case where the husband may have a condition impairing his ability to read his wife's emotions, it is unjust to hold him entirely at fault. Over and over, Martin is told that he needs to change in order for the marriage to work, but Louisa doesn't provide him with a pathway to expressing emotions Martin has no way of voicing, nor is Louisa ever severely challenged for her own contributions to their marriage's problems.

Eventually, Martin and Louisa reconcile, but the central issue affecting Martin's interactions is completely sidestepped. In "The Doctor Is Out" (S7E8), the two come to an understanding, but there is not any real depth to a better comprehension over why Martin is the man he is. In this conversation, they say:

LOUISA. I think I've made a terrible mistake. I think I'm a bit obsessed with everyone having to be normal. People aren't, are they?

MARTIN. No.

LOUISA. I'm not, you're not. You, you're unusual. Everyone said that maybe you just left. I knew you wouldn't let me down, the one person who never has. I just knew you wouldn't, I just knew in my heart.

MARTIN. You know I'm never going to change how I feel about you.

LOUISA. I don't want that.

MARTIN. I've tried. I've really tried, but it just makes things worse.

LOUISA. Can we go home now?

It is a reconciliation, but there is no real comprehension. The writers have managed to resolve the strain in the marriage that they introduced, but the episode sidesteps the question of why Martin is the way he is. Louisa has made the journey to accept, but the "everybody's different" remark minimizes the difficulties that neuroatypical people face. By this scene, Louisa has gained the *attitude* necessary to create a better relationship with her husband, but not the *understanding* necessary to address the root cause of the problems that dampen her enthusiasm for the marriage.

Moving on, the character of Christopher Boone in *The Curious Incident of the Dog in the Night-Time* has long been a controversial one in the autistic community, provoking both powerfully positive and negative responses. Reactions as to whether his characterization is reflective of many people with autism, or if he simply embodies many stereotypes about people on the spectrum vary widely, and to focus on the contrasting critical reactions of Christopher Boone might fill up a book in itself. Here, I wish to focus simply on generalized criticisms of Christopher for his alleged lack of empathy.[*]

These criticisms of Christopher's often focus on perceived shortcomings in his personality, though such assessments are based more on his characterization in the novel. This leads to the question: Why isn't he warmer or kinder or more sympathetic towards others? Why are his comments so often unfeeling and insensitive? His alleged lack of sympathy for his classmates is often held against him. But these criticisms of Christopher Boone essentially condemn him for his conditions. If autism spectrum disorder is indeed a factor in his mental mindset, then his brain is programmed in such a way that he has extreme difficulty understanding how other people respond and why they act as they do.

It is unfair to ask a person with certain forms of autism to demonstrate certain levels of understanding regarding other people. Once again, autism does not equate to an inherent ability to feel empathy, but it does mean that an autistic person may have serious difficulties understanding why someone else might find a comment offensive, or find another person's actions frustrating. The autistic may be able to form better connections with others over time, but this often requires support and guidance from trusted sources. Christopher never received the full level of support that he needed.

---

[*] I have read many of these criticisms on autism-related Internet message boards, and I am deliberately avoiding naming names of critics so as not to create a one-sided debate or to target individuals who I do not know personally for their opinions.

Throughout the play, Christopher is held to a standard that he has not been trained to follow. Often, caring parents are the primary force for teaching their autistic children how to respond to others, but though the Boones clearly love their son, there are strong clues throughout the play that Mr. and Mrs. Boone are both deeply flawed people whose personal issues may have prevented them from providing much-needed guidance. Ed Boone clearly has anger management problems, as evidenced by his outbursts and his act of violence against a helpless dog. In comparison, Judy Boone went for a disturbingly long time without hearing from her son. She did send him letters which were intercepted by her husband, but her excuse that she just thought that Christopher was angry at her and would resume contact when he was ready is either naïve or self-serving. Nothing was stopping her from calling or making a visit or asking some third party to check in on Christopher and ask him about the situation. If one is being cynical, one could argue that Judy was just enjoying a break from having to care for her special needs son, and instead of worrying about his lack of communication with her, simply decided avoidance was the best strategy, ignoring the potential emotional trauma that her son faced. Shortly after their reunion, Judy reminisces amount a terrible meltdown that Christopher once had, and though she does not castigate him for his emotional outburst, she does bring up the fact that he accidentally injured her, and in much of her dialogue throughout the play, she puts heavy stress on how Christopher's difficulties affect her. Parenting children with special needs can be a challenge, and caregivers deserve sympathy as much as the children they look after, but Judy's approach to parenting, from what is shown in the play, often focuses on placating Christopher's intense emotional outbursts, and she is not shown attempting to teach Christopher how to improve his interpersonal skills.

Not only is Christopher's family life inadequate to the task of teaching him how to interact with others, but his schooling is similarly flawed. Christopher goes to a school for young people with special needs, but it's indicated that many of his classmates are severely developmentally disabled, and that his level of functionality and intelligence far exceeds any of his peers. Though the play does not point this out directly, Christopher's mindset has caused him to fall into the cracks of the educational system. His issues interacting with others mean that he would probably not fit in at a regular school filled with neurotypical young people. However, he also does not fit in with his other special needs classmates. The teachers at Christopher's school are trained to deal with young people with communication difficulties, continence problems, and an inability to be self-reliant. Christopher's exceptional mathematical abilities might have gone wasted because his school was not equipped to give him a test. The school was more concerned about the fallout of setting a precedent by giving Christopher supposed "special treatment" by allowing him to take a national mathematics examination. It was only his father's pressure that made it possible for Christopher to take the exam. The character of Siobhan (Niamh Cusack) is often described as a kindly mentor for Christopher, but in the scene where Mr. Boone demands that Christopher be allowed to take the examination, she's the voice of an unfeeling bureaucracy, parroting lines about equal treatment, and bolstering a system designed to prevent Christopher from succeeding or advancing.

Once again, if one uses a sympathetic lens to take Christopher's side, it's unfair to view him as an unfeeling person, and it is much more just to view him as a victim of a culture that is not equipped to accommodate someone who is mentally wired like he is. This is not meant to defend his occasionally offensive behavior, but it should be stressed that Christopher ought not to be blamed for his behavior and attitudes, as he does not have the ability to instinctually know how to respond in certain situations. No one would blame a teenager for not knowing a foreign language or understanding calculus without proper education. Likewise, it is unfair to chastise Christopher for his social ineptitude when he has not received adequate guidance regarding his behavior.

Many people think the treatment for autistic reactions is aversion therapy. Provide enough exposure to whatever affects the autistic person negatively, and eventually that person will become desensitized to it. That may help in some instances, but in many cases, such supposed treatment for autistic reactions leads to reactions closer to sufferers of peanut allergies or celiac disease. Repeated exposure to the allergen does not build tolerance, but often the opposite is true. Increased exposure can mean heightened sensitivity. That is why for some people with autism, more frequent social activity can improve interpersonal skills, whereas for others, a similar program of interaction can lead to exhaustion and reluctance to deal with future social situations. Heightened exposure only makes the situation worse in some instances.

In all of these portrayals, the characters are routinely blamed for their actions and attitudes, but those who castigate them, whether they are fictional characters or real-life critics, would benefit from a more sympathetic viewpoint. This is not meant to use autism as an excuse to absolve these characters of all blame, but it is a reminder that preconceived notions amongst the neurotypical may misinterpret autistic characteristics and unfairly view struggling with uncaringness. It also illustrates how undiagnosed autism, a misinformed or undereducated public, and a failure to receive helpful treatment and teaching, may leave autistic people struggling to survive in an uncomfortable world.

CONCLUSION
Personal Perspectives, Connections, and Suggestions for Improvement

Aside from the introductory chapters, I have mostly tried to keep myself out of this analysis. This was the correct decision for the lion's share of this study, but as part of the goal of this critical inquiry was to evaluate the dramatic depictions of autism, in order to do so effectively, they must be compared to real-life people with autism, and the only autistic mind that I can say I know thoroughly is my own.

To reiterate the point that I have made many times before, each autistic mind is unique, and one depiction that is a perfect replica of one autistic person's mind may be radically dissimilar from another's. There is no such thing as a "typical" neuroatypical mind. Some people with autism may see themselves in a dramatization portraying someone on the spectrum. Other autistic individuals may consider the same production to be a caricature or even a complete distortion of their personal experiences.

Over the past several years, I have participated in numerous online discussion groups for both autism and mystery entertainment, and though none of the forums in which I participate combine the two, there has been some overlap between the two topics, as some of my correspondents on the autism forums discussed the protagonists of the crime dramas they watched, and noted how similarly these characters mirrored their own mental processes and social experiences. Meanwhile, a few of the mystery discussion forums, on multiple occasions have suggested that a television detective is on the spectrum, even though the matter is never brought up on the show.

And this is why I wrote this book. I wanted to address a growing controversy in the autistic community in a way that would be accessible to as many people as possible, whether they had any background in neurological issues or not, and I also wanted to appeal to mystery fans with an interest in analyzing some of their favorite detectives, In addition, I aimed to understand why entertainment industry creatives have, over the course of the twenty-first century, both created so many prominent characters with autistic attributes, but also avoided labelling these detectives with a definite diagnosis of autism. Why are the only characters to be openly and consistently described as autistic the most recently introduced ones in this study, and why has the entertainment industry been so traditionally reluctant to provide these characters with a diagnosis? In response to these questions, I have no direct insight into the writers' rooms. I have access only to what has been shown on screens.

Once again, except in cases where one of the fictional sleuths discussed here is expressly diagnosed with autism, I am not arguing that any of the characters definitely has autism. The point is that each of these characters has attributes that are *suggestive* of autism, and the goal is to use these characters as examples that viewers on the autism spectrum can employ to compare and contrast to their own perspectives, and use them as tools to communicate their own personal mental make-ups. To reiterate, between and a quarter and a third of the characters analyzed in this study are borderline to the point that a reasonable argument can be made that the characters have only a very mild form of autism, or other conditions or simple personality make-ups that mirror some aspects of autism.

I should stress that in nearly every case, I'm a fan – often a big fan – of the shows and actors discussed here, and any criticisms I may have levelled are never directed towards the actors' performances. Ultimately, my major complaint with many of these series is that the creators and writers often broach the idea that a character has autism, and then never bother to address it. Most of these characters never receive professional help to resolve any challenges they may face – they are largely left to handle everything on their own. Any psychological treatment the character receives may address some emotional or social issue, but by and large, the shows dance around the major issue, which means that any help the characters receive is not as effective as it might be.

People who watch these portrayals may be dispirited by watching entertainment that depicts individuals who think and act like them, and then have no recourse for help with their difficulties. Overwhelmingly, the message – consciously or unconsciously – being pushed by these shows is that the only way for autistic people to survive and succeed in their career goals is to press forward, grit your teeth, and bear through any difficulties, and your idiosyncrasies will draw mockery and suspicion from many people no matter what you do. If you can't mirror neurotypical behavior, you're out of luck. Sometimes, like in *Sherlock*, one can push back with a similar attitude, but that does not create understanding, only resentment. The best you can hope for is to have a supportive collection of friends and family members to help you power through. Only in the most recent series, *Astrid et Raphaëlle* and *Extraordinary Attorney Woo*, are unconventional tactics and strategies utilized to help the autistic titular characters. In real life, people with autism are commonly told just to "stop being weird" or that they're being annoying, as if the reactions of those around them are more important than the internal anguish that the autistic are struggling to survive.

And part of this is due in part to the fact that many popular culture depictions of autism only deal with externals.

Speech patterns, movements, and social awkwardness are easier to portray than the internal turmoil that autistic people deal with on a daily basis. And part of the reason is that realistic dramatic presentations can only only certain aspects of events such as an autism meltdown. When portrayed on-screen, viewers can see screaming, crying, and jerky movements, and interpret them as a kind of temper tantrum. Perhaps a touch, or a sound sets off the autistic character, and the casual neurotypical viewer may look at this reaction and conclude that the character is throwing a fit because everything isn't exactly as he or she wants it to be. It's fussiness rather than a reaction to being overwhelmed. A UK video produced by the National Autistic Society titled "What If We Could Change This?" showed a little boy being led through a shopping mall, and over the course of a minute and a half, viewers would see him responding to flickering lights, squirted perfume, loud noises, and it culminates in a meltdown. Neurotypical people just see ordinary surroundings. People with certain forms of autism see a constant bombardment of stimuli that drain their concentration and focus. At the end of the video, the little boy gives a brief voiceover, saying "I'm not naughty. I'm autistic." Even in adulthood, these reactions, like uncontrollable tears, shaking, and screaming, can assault an autistic person with devastating strength. To the unsympathetic and uninformed neurotypical person, this is childish behavior that should be shamed and suppressed. And it's not entirely due to a lack of empathy. It's driven by insufficient understanding.

One of my deepest hopes is that many other people with autism can find ways to describe their mental processes in a visual manner, so as to convey them better to others. When watching the performances of Downey and Cumberbatch, I was stunned because both productions replicated my own thought processes on-screen. From childhood, I have anticipated actions and reactions in visual and audial forms in my mind, exactly as depicted in the Downey films. The visual predictions of future actions can be so vivid that sometimes I can be temporarily uncertain whether I have actually performed those actions or if I simply thought about them very intensely. Additionally, when observing people and surroundings, I commonly add my own annotations to what I see just like in *Sherlock*, superimposing what I think upon what I see, though the notes I create in my mind are not just text, but images, audio, and video as well.

In future television shows and continuing ones, it would be helpful to see less coyness about naming neurological conditions, and to not just portray mannerisms and quirks, but to delve deeper into how openly autistic people knowingly deal with their challenges. For me, the vision of the autistic sleuth is an ideal to aspire to rather than a limiting stereotype.

There are a lot of people with autism who need additional help with ordinary functioning and improving their communication skills. It is my hope that this book can in some small way assist people on the spectrum and those who care about them. I will say it again. A lot of people with autism have reactions that are radically different from mine and the characters depicted here. But by exploring these examples, maybe other people with autism can find their own voices through comparing and contrasting.

The critical point is that I am trying to overcome any limitations placed on me by autism. At the same time, I have no desire whatsoever to have my autistic tendencies removed or even mitigated. After my intense migraine attacks, my autistic reactions were dialed down to the lowest levels of my life, but I lost most of my creative and analytical abilities. I wasn't freaking out at the slightest touch or unpleasant smell, but I was miserable and I felt as if I was mentally straitjacketed. When my brain healed, everything returned. Adrian Monk often refers to his abilities as "a blessing... and a curse." I often feel the same way.

After reading this book, I hope that people with autism can use the discussions and analysis appearing here as a template for explaining what they're feeling – even if they reject my premises and believe that entirely different styles, approaches, topics of study should be used in future analysis. I believe that the pathways to helping people understand their own minds, abilities, and how to help themselves communicate and succeed in any field they wish to the best of their abilities. I hope that therapists and teachers who work with the autistic may be inspired to incorporate dramatic depictions of autism into their work. I do not know if my self-taught therapy methods of using Arthur Conan Doyle, G.K. Chesterton, and Agatha Christie books to help me understand how other people think will work with many other people, but I would be very interested to see if anyone else could find success using comparable methods. Additionally, I hope that writers strive harder to understand what autism is and reconsider their previous hesitancy to diagnose characters.

On numerous occasions, I've heard a neurotypical person say that autism can be treated through therapy or social conditioning. Certainly such treatments can help with the interpersonal problems resulting from autism, but there's much more to it than that. A lot of these declarations are based on faulty assumptions, that improvement in social interactions means a decrease in involuntary physical and emotional responses to stimuli. The problem with a lot of supposed "therapies" is that the goal is to turn an autistic person into a neurotypical person, or at least make an autistic person capable of acting neurotypical. This approach does not teach people with autism to be themselves, but instead, these tactics try to turn them into an uncomfortable, twisted version of themselves where every interaction is inauthentic, and excruciating stress is placed upon the arbitrary approval of others.

    Perhaps the exploding trend of the autistic sleuth happened because awareness of autism led screenwriters to decide that they wanted to incorporate an "interesting quirk" into their characterization. Over time, it's become a cultural phenomenon that deserves closer scrutiny and discussion. I don't know what the future will hold for this trend, but it will be interesting to me to see how future writers and actors portray autism on-screen, in the crime genre and beyond.

Appendix: 12 Things to Know About Parishioners with Autism

I wrote this pamphlet as part of an endeavor to help the Archdiocese of Milwaukee reach out to parishioners with autism, but the messages in it are not limited to any single group, religious or otherwise.

1) What is Autism?

Autism spectrum disorders are neurological conditions that affect how people think and respond to certain stimuli. People with autism can have serious trouble connecting with others and communicating. Their behavior is often involuntary. Some people with autism live independent lives; others need lifelong care and assistance. It's a diverse condition thataffects people in a wide variety of ways, and an approach to help one autistic person may not work for another autistic person.

We don't know the causes of autism for certain, but previous theories that it was caused by vaccines or neglectful mothering have been debunked.

Autism is NOT consistent amongst everybody who has it. There's a saying that "if you've met one person with autism… you've met one person with autism." Autism manifests itself differently in different people, and the severity and nature of one's reactions differs from person to person, and each person on the autistic spectrum may react differently depending on the time.

2) Autism is not mental illness or neurosis.

Autism is NOT a form of mental illness, and it cannot be "cured." It is a different form of neurological wiring, and though people with autism may need special care and helped by trained psychologists, autism isn't something that can be "fixed." Many autistic people can, however, learn how to cope with their condition better with proper care and assistance.
Sometimes autistic children's difficulties fade as they grow older, but not always. Sometimes problems undulate over the course of a lifetime.

It must be noted that autistic people can develop depression, anxiety, and other forms of actual mental illness just like everybody else. Often, feeling isolated and misunderstood canlead to depression. Unfortunately, the brain chemistry of autistic people is often (not always) different from neurotypical people, and certain autistic people respond differently to some medications than others. The side effects can be intense because the medicines may affect the autistic brain in a radically different manner from the average neurotypical person.

3) **Discomfort is often unavoidable.**

Just as no one can hope to live in a completely perfect world, regrettably, no matter how much effort one puts into helping the autistic, there's no way to create a totally perfect environment that will leave autistic people completely unaffected. Sometimes the best one can do isn't enough. Often it takes trial and error to figure out what works and what doesn't for each specific person. Explaining that this is a learning process for all people involved can be a respectful approach to guidance.

4) **"Acting out" is not necessarily deliberate misbehavior**

To be clear, autistic children can misbehave, but often their meltdowns and attempts to cope with situations that overstimulate and upset them can be misconstrued. Autistic meltdowns can be mistaken for temper tantrums.

A UK campaign to raise awareness about autistic children's reactions used the tagline, "I'm not naughty. I'm autistic." In these commercials, little sensory triggers such as the scent of perfume, the flash of florescent lighting, constant noise, and being surrounded by strangers caused an autistic child to collapse in tears and screams. This point underscores the need for greater understanding of the autistic experience.

5) **Change can be traumatic**

We hear the phrase "change is good" a lot. This is not necessarily the case for autistic people, who are often so overwhelmed by their surroundings that they cling to consistency in order to keep their moorings and maintain a sense of stability in a world that seems to shift under their feet constantly. A substitute teacher, a changed hairstyle, a different location, or even a slight disruption in the usual routine can cause an autistic child to respond negatively.

This does *not* mean that everything should be kept as static as possible to accommodate the autistic. It simply means that an upcoming change, like a switch in personnel, a move, or rescheduling can provoke distress. Letting the autistic child in question know about the upcoming change as soon as possible, and explaining that it's unavoidable but how helpful their flexibility on the matter is, can mitigate the situation.

6) **Mimicking "neurotypical" behavior is not always possible or even desirable.**

It can be exhausting, even crushing, to pretend to be someone that you are not. Pressuring autistic people, especially children, to act in a manner described as "normal" can be devastating. While guidance on forming friendships and other personal interactions is often necessary and appreciated, forcing autistic people to speak or move or respond in a mannerthat feels unnatural to them can have harmful effects. Just as trying to correct a limp with ametal brace that is so restrictive it causes muscle damage and torn skin is unhealthy, so is compelling the autistic to adopt a neurological and behavioral corset.

Ultimately, the goal for working with autistic people is not to eliminate their autistic tendencies or to train them to suppress their atypical speech and movement habits.
Autistic people should be helped to interact with others and better understand their own reactions and brain chemistry. The goal should be to help autistic people succeed in life andconnect better with others while still remaining wholly themselves.

7) People with autism often have very strong moral codes, affecting reactions

Autistic people may enjoy the structure of rules, leading to anger towards those who break them. This can lead to condemnatory behavior, and it can also cause outrage if people aren't "properly punished" (in their eyes) for infractions. This can cause autistic children to be seen as "snitches" by their peers, and adults need to be very cautious about gossiping about other adults' alleged transgressions within the hearing of autistic children– this might
lead to some embarrassing confrontations later.

There is no easy solution to this, but it can really help if autistic children have a trusted adult they can turn to in order to discuss their concerns and feelings.

8) **Logical answers to questions help.**

"Just because" just doesn't work as an explanation. Calm and rational responses, which always show respect to those asking the questions, are more helpful. Sometimes different approaches are necessary to discuss complex topics, ranging from academic subjects to
religious matters to social and personal issues. Also, one shouldn't be afraid to say that one needs further time and research in order to answer a question more thoroughly and accurately.

9) **Discomfort or unease expressed by the autistic should not be taken personally.**

Some autistic people, especially children, may not be aware of the effects that their actions have on other people. They may be distracted by other stimuli, such as noises in the background, something they consider to be "out of order," or even feeling discomfort in the chair in which they are sitting. They may not be able to look others in the eye, or if they are feeling overwhelmed, their ability to communicate may be harmed. Sometimes, some autistic people may feel the need to leave a social situation abruptly, because they feel sick or otherwise highly uncomfortable. Often, these actions are not meant to be rude, but are meant as a means of self-protection.

Sometimes offense may be given unintentionally. The important thing is to differentiate between the *deliberate* causing of offense and the *inadvertent* causing of offense.

It is often said that the autistic have a poor sense of empathy. In many cases, this is radically unfair and serves to marginalize and even denigrate the autistic. A better description of many autistic people is that *it is more challenging for them to understand how other people think and react differently from them*. That does not mean they are incapable of learning how other people feel and respond, nor does it mean that they do not care. It simply means that often, more effort and innovative methods, ranging from in-depth discussions to reading fiction or watching movies about comparative people and situations, is needed to help the autistic understand other people's thoughts and feelings.

10) Autistic children may need extra care and protection.

Just because the autistic can have heightened awareness of their surroundings, that does not mean that they are conscious of all of the potential dangers threatening them. They may be lost in thought or distracted by stimuli, leaving them unaware of certain threats, like a cyclist or a car coming in their direction. Furthermore, autistic children may be less likely to spot the dangerous attentions of predators. Unsympathetic teachers or misguided therapists can also have damaging effects of autistic children.

11) **Autism affects many aspects of Mass attendance and other aspects of religious observance.**

Attending Mass can be very stressful for autistic people. The crowds, the sounds, the smells… every sensory experience has an effect on the autistic brain, and it can lead to physiological and mental consequences ranging from meltdowns and "Asperger's
moments" to internal distress. Some autistic people may feel or believe to feel heightened contact with the supernatural at mass, and this can lead to intense reactions.

The overwhelming nature of it all causes many autistic people to abandon religious practices and never come back. Understanding the physical and psychological reactions that contribute to this phenomenon may be able to change the issue. Some autistic people also feel like something's spiritually wrong with them, and there may be despair or resentment over not being able to take part in church activities, and anticipating events such as Sunday mass can be very stressful. Often understanding *what* is happening inside one's head can mean a great deal of difference to an autistic person's emotional, psychological, and spiritual well-being.

12) **Special accommodations may need to be made. Not everything can (or should) be changed to help autistic people, but small, separate steps may be taken. Special "autism friendly" masses, or one-on-one conversations can help.**

Unfortunately, there's no way to remove all of the potential stimuli that can overwhelm an autistic person, but there are various ways that situations may be helped. Crowds, sounds, and smells can be critical problems. Occasional "autism friendly" masses with fewer people, disconnected loudspeakers, and limited incense may be more helpful for autistic children, and often faith formation is easier in one-on-one or small group discussions, without being surrounded by their peers.

"Autism friendly" does not mean "one size fits all." Talking to people, especially children, about what does and doesn't help them is the only way to find out how they can feel more comfortable (or at least less overwhelmed). Unfortunately, no one knows what will help until something's been tried.

CONCLUSION
Autistic people are members of the Body of Christ who want to belong and contribute to church life, just like anybody else. They may just need a little more assistance and understanding than most people.

BIBLIOGRAPHY

Articles

Budryk, Zack. "The Evolution of the 'Mildly Autistic Super-Detective.'" CrimeReads. https://crimereads.com/the-evolution-of-the-mildly-autistic-super-detective/ (accessed February 15, 2024).

Loftis, Sonya Freeman. "The Autistic Detective: Sherlock Holmes and His Legacy." *Disability Studies Quarterly*. https://dsq-sds.org/index.php/dsq/article/view/3728/3791 (accessed February 15, 2024).

"Neurodivergent Representation in Sherlock Holmes." The Nineteenth-Century Novel. https://blogs.dickinson.edu/19thcennovel/2022/11/19/neurodivergent-representation-in-sherlock-holmes/ (accessed February 15, 2024).

Rossi, Carey. "The Autistic Brain." *Psycom*. https://www.psycom.net/autism-brain-differences (accessed February 15, 2024).

Books

Baron-Cohen, Simon. *The Pattern Seekers: How Autism Drives Human Invention*. New York City, U.S.A.: Basic Books, 2020.

Donvan, John and Caren Zucker. *In a Different Key: The Story of Autism*. New York City, U.S.A.: Crown Publishing Group, 2016.

Doyle, Arthur Conan. *The Complete Sherlock Holmes*. New York City, U.S.A.: Doubleday, 1930;

Grandin, Temple. *Visual Thinking: The Hidden Gifts of People Who Think in Pictures, Patterns, and Abstractions.* New York City, U.S.A.: Riverhead Books, 2022.

Grandin, Temple with Richard Panek. *The Autistic Brain: Helping Different Kinds of Minds Succeed.* Boston, U.S.A.: Mariner Books, 2014.

Filmed Stage Productions
The Curious Incident of the Dog in the Night-Time (2012)
Death Note: The Musical (2015)

Movies
Death Note (2006)
Death Note 2: The Last Name (2006)
Death Note 3: L: Change the World (2008)
The Girl in the Spider's Web (2018)
The Girl with the Dragon Tattoo (2009)
The Girl with the Dragon Tattoo (2011)
The Millennium Trilogy (The Girl with the Dragon Tattoo (2009), The Girl who Played with Fire (2009), The Girl Who Kicked the Hornet's Nest (2009))
The Night Clerk (2020)
Sherlock Holmes (2009)
Sherlock Holmes: A Game of Shadows (2011)

Online Sources
The Internet Movie Database (www.imdb.com)
National Autistic Society. "What If We Could Change This?" YouTube.
https://www.youtube.com/watch?v=6_pyskoO9X4)
(accessed February 15, 2024).

Reilly, Elaine. ""*Professor T*" Star Ben Miller: "I Was Born to Play This Part." Whattowatch. https://www.whattowatch.com/features/professor-t-star-ben-miller-i-was-born-to-play-this-part (accessed February 15, 2024).

The Vile Eye. "Analyzing Evil: Dexter Morgan." YouTube. https://www.youtube.com/watch?v=30PINcn4lFg (accessed February 15, 2024).

Television Series
24 (2001-2010)
24: Live Another Day (2014)
Astrid et Raphaëlle (also released as "Astrid" and "Bright Minds") (2019– Present)
Bones (2005-2017)
The Bridge (2013-2014)
The Bridge (Bron/Broen) (2011-2018)
The Brief (2004-2005)
Chasing Shadows (2014)
Community (2009-2015)
Criminal Minds (2005-Present)
CSI: Crime Scene Investigation (2000-2015)
Detective Sweet (2016)
Dexter (2006-2013)
Dexter: New Blood (2021-2022)
Doc Martin (2004-2022)
Elementary (2012-2019)
Elsbeth (2024-Present)
Extraordinary Attorney Woo (2022-Present)
Hannibal (2013-2015)
IQ 246: The Cases of a Royal Genius (2016)
King & Maxwell (2013)

Law & Order: Criminal Intent (2001–2011)
Law & Order: Special Victims Unit (1999–Present)
Law & Order: Trial By Jury (2005)
Miss Sherlock (2018)
Monk (2002–2009)
Mr. Mercedes (2017–2019)
Murdoch Mysteries (2008–Present)
The No. 1 Ladies' Detective Agency (2008)
The Outsider (2020)
Professor T (2019–Present)
Queens of Mystery (2019–Present)
Sherlock (2010-2017)
The Shield (2002-2008)
The Tunnel (2013-2018)

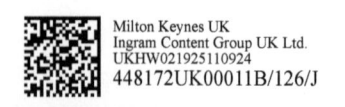

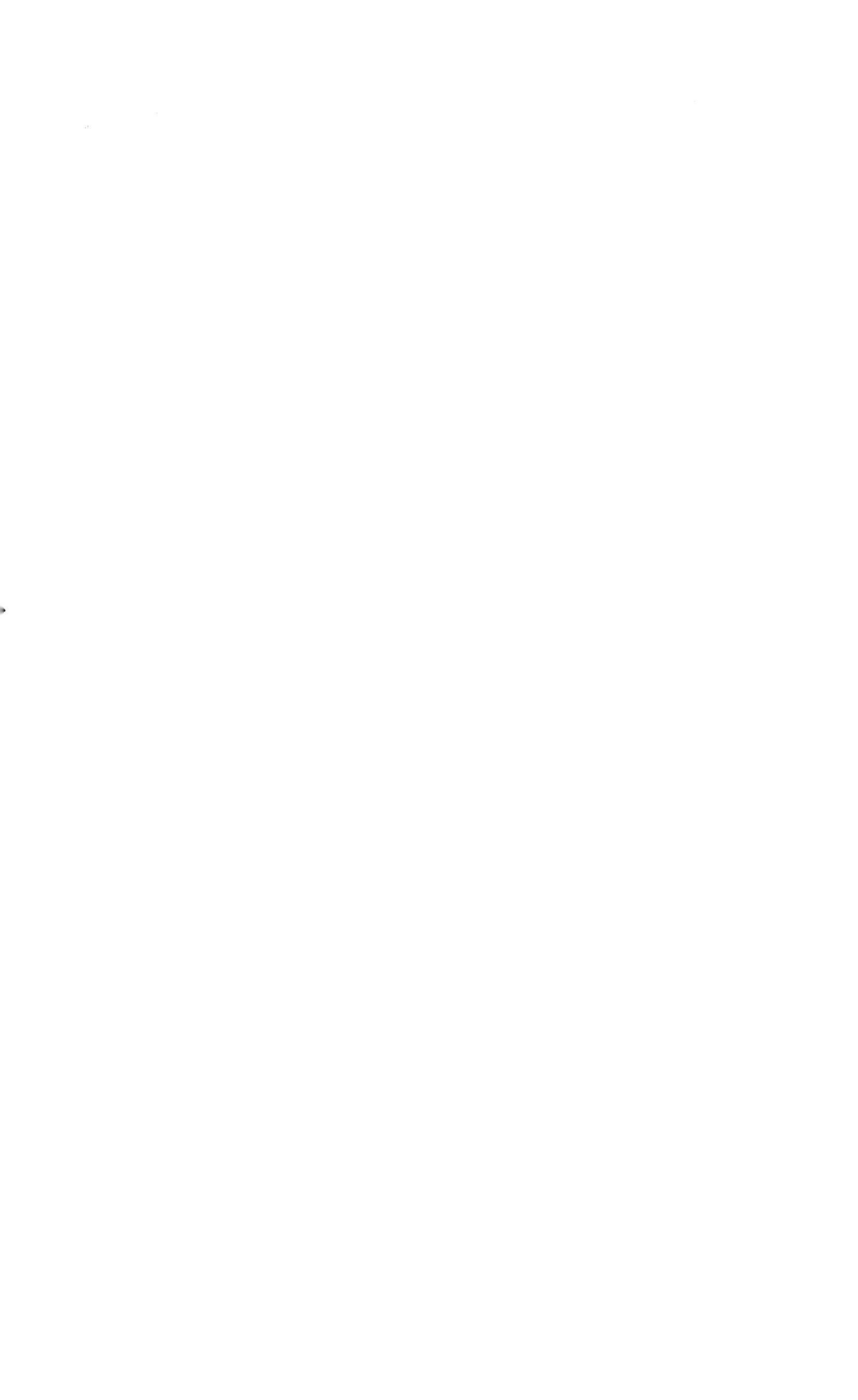